Predatory Lending

Toxic Credit in the Global Inner City

An Afterword to Predatory Bender, *A Story of Subprime Finance*

by Matthew Lee

INNER
CITY
PRESS
1919 Washington Ave
Bronx NY 10457
InnerCityPress.org

ISBN 0-9740244-1-4   Printed in the United States of America

Library of Congress Control Number: 2003111283
(among with *Predatory Bender: A Story of Subprime Finance*)

Library of Congress Cataloging-in-Publication Data
is available from the publisher upon request

About the Author: Matthew Lee is a public interest lawyer, growing out
of community-controlled housing battles in the South Bronx of New
York City stretching back to 1987. He has published analysis pieces in
New York Newsday, American Banker, City Limits and elsewhere. He
has been involved in seeking accountability from banks and other
corporations since the early 1990s, and now does this work globally
through the Fair Finance Watch and its Human Rights Enforcement
Project.

Cover design by Janine-Marie Boulad.

For information on Inner City Press reading group guides, as well as ordering
for use in educational institutions, contact editor@innercitypress.org. A portion
of the sales from each copy of this book goes to the Fair Finance Watch, which
advocates for consumers' and human rights.

I want to join Fair Finance Watch and receive a 10% discount on this and
all subsequent orders. Enclosed is my contribution of: $100 - $50 - $30

Name
Address
City/State/Zip
Daytime Phone
E-mail

Make check or money order payable to:

Inner City Press, PO Box 580188, Mt. Carmel Station, Bronx NY 10458

1.

Borrowing money is a way of life and death. To buy a home or start a small business, to build a dam or fight a war: it all requires finance. It is doled out by banks and their casino called Wall Street. In alleyways from The Bronx to Beijing there are loan sharks as well, offering fast cash and then collecting with baseball bats and foreclosures. That the World Bank and the International Monetary Fund do this as well will be explored later. We start with transactions in their simplest form: two thousand dollars, say, to buy needed household goods.

In the United States in the first decade of the 21st century there are many storefronts offering such loans. Some are old -- Household Finance and its sister Beneficial, for example -- and some are newer-fangled, like CitiFinancial. Both offer credit at rates over thirty percent. The business is booming: the spreads, Wall Street says, are too good to pass up. Citibank pays under five percent interest on the deposits it collects. Its affiliated loan sharks charge four times that rate, even for loans secured by the borrower's home. It's a can't-miss proposition. Even if the economy goes South they can take and resell the collateral. The business is global: the Hong Kong & Shanghai Banking Corporation, now HSBC, wants to export it to the eighty-plus countries in which it has a retail presence. Institutional investors love the business model and investment banks securitize the loans. These fancy terms will be defined as we proceed.

The root, however, the fodder on which the whole pyramid rests, is the solitary customer at what's called the point of sale. It's a magic trick, really, perhaps a form of bad religion, the way the points and fees can be added to the money that's lent. CitiFinancial and Household Finance both suggest that insurance is needed. This they serve in a number of flavors -- credit life and credit disability, credit unemployment and property insurance -- but in almost all cases, it is included in the loans and interest is charged on it. It's called "single premium" -- instead of paying each month for coverage, you pay in advance with money on which you pay interest. If you choose to refinance, you will not get a refund. It is money down the drain, but at the point-of-sale it often goes unnoticed.

2.

Take, for example, the purchase of furniture. A bedroom set might cost two thousand dollars. The sign says Easy Credit, sometimes spelled E-Z. The furniture man does not manage these accounts. For this he turns to CitiFinancial, to HFC or perhaps to Wells Fargo. While the Federal Reserve lends money to banks at below five percent, these bank-affiliates charge twenty or thirty or forty percent. You will have insurance on your furniture: to protect you, they say, from having it repossessed if you die or become unemployed. Before the debt is discharged, dead or alive, you will have paid more than the list-price of a luxury car or a crypt with a doorman.

Midway you'll be approached with a sweet-sounding offer: if you'll put up your home as collateral, your rate can be lowered and the term be extended. A twenty-year mortgage, fixed or adjustable. The rate will be high and the rules not disclosed. For example: if you satisfy the loan too quickly, you'll be charged a pre-payment penalty. Or, you'll pay slowly and then be asked to pay more, in what's called a balloon. If you can't, that's okay: they knew you couldn't. The goal is to refinance your loan and charge you yet more points and fees.

In prior centuries, this was called debt peonage. Today it is the fate of the so-called subprime serf. Fully twenty percent of American households are described as subprime. But half of the people who get subprime loans could have paid normal rates, according to Fannie Mae and Beltway authorities. Outside it's the law of the jungle; the only rule is Buyer Beware. But this is easier for some people than others.

Why would a person overpay by so much? In the nation's low-income neighborhoods, sometimes called ghettos or, in a more poetic euphemism, the inner city, there's a lack of bank branches. In the late 20th century, many financial institutions left the 'hood in the lurch. They refused to lend money; they refused to write insurance policies. This is called redlining, since in one apocryphal case the bank drew on a map a line in red pen around the neighborhood to be avoided. The South Bronx was one; so too Chicago's South Side and Watts in Los Angeles. In the District of Columbia, Anacostia and Southeast were allowed to go to seed. The city of East St. Louis nearly disappeared amid weeds and empty buildings. This is redlining, a major explanation for homelessness.

But the postmodern twist is for the same banks which left to return with loan shark affiliates. It's one thing to sell cups of water for one hundred dollars in a desert. But when the seller is the one who slashed and burned the land, creating the need, it is something else. In the New Testament, Jesus whipped the money changers. The Koran, going further, prohibits the lending of money at interest. But today's new religion is stock-price and it's measured in quarters. In the absence of law there is only the jungle.

3.

Those who profit from loan sharks are sometimes far away. Take, for example, the Lehman Brothers firm. It does not have any storefronts, in Anacostia or The Bronx. What it does is provide money, in the form of warehouse loans, to the companies that best-know this downscale market. There was one called First Alliance; it charged rates over fifteen percent. It got exposed in the press and then sued by the government. The court fights continued, now against Lehman. The money lent by First Alliance all comes from Wall Street. Lehman provides a line of credit, and then buys the high-rate mortgages just after they're made. Lehman doesn't keep them -- it "pools" them and rates them and sells them in pieces. A hedge fund, say, can buy an interest-only strip. Another company called the trustee -- Deutsche Bank is big in this business -- collects the money that's owed on the loans and funnels the interest portion to those who bought the I/O strip. One could also buy the principal (yes, the "P/O") -- it all depends on one's guess about interest rates and the economy. This is high-stakes poker for well-paid card sharks. But the chips that they trade are poorer people's homes. This is securitization.

There are other roles for Wall Street: the analysis of the debt and equity securities of subprime lenders, and merger advisory work when the companies are sold. HSBC's mad dash to buy Household, for example, was a marriage designed by Goldman Sachs and Morgan Stanley, with some Doctor Ruth advice also provided by Felix Rohatyn. This last was the man who is said to have saved New York. Now he plays matchmaker for a loan shark and a redliner. Such counseling is lucrative. The law firms on the deal include Cleary Gottlieb and Wachtell Lipton, and later Milbank Tweed. More on these anon. [*See* Chapterette 34.]

4.

There are, of course, opponents. Consumer watchdogs and community-based groups, and, seemingly in a different sphere, class action lawyers. First Alliance was sued by just such a wolf pack. State attorneys general also play a role: just prior to HSBC's bear hug, Household settled with states for half a billion dollars. Citigroup, given the political juice it enjoys or enjoyed, paid half that amount, to six times the victims. These settlements, in the language of Wall Street, are a cost of doing business. At most, Citigroup pays back sixty cents on each dollar it stole. In exchange it gets a waiver: the people accepting the settlement checks cannot sue Citi again. Worse, if or when Citigroup forecloses on their homes, the settlees cannot raise as a defense the fraud of the loan. That sin's been purged, through the mystery of a nationwide class action the filing of which Citigroup itself solicited. [*See* Chapterette 21.]

If it's a regulated business, where then are the regulators? One of them's the same cabal which sets the rates: the Federal Reserve. The Fed has jurisdiction over all bank holding companies, including Citigroup, Morgan Chase and Wells Fargo. Each owns a subprime lender. But the Fed, at least under Greenspan, has had its eye on bigger, more ideological quarry. As Atlas Shrugged, Mr. Greenspan raised his brow. He believes in free markets, while setting the rules of the game with his rates. When friends of his fail -- take Long Term Capital Management, co-run by ex-Fed Dave Mullins -- he can arrange some new loans. The subprime borrower, however, is on his or her own. When Citigroup bought Associates First Capital in late 2000, the Fed required nothing, not even a public hearing. Subsequently the Fed said it would examine CitiFinancial -- and then dragged this on for nearly two years. There were foreclosures; there was crying. But the Federal Reserve's temple, white marble in front of the Mall, is sound-proofed.

5.

For the Fed it's enough if banks *say* they have safeguards. Citigroup, for example, says it does mystery shopping. It tests itself, which the Fed likes to hear. But the test's answer code was passed out in advance. Employees were told in what months they'd be tested, and what the topics were. Not surprisingly, there was a very high pass rate. The list of the failures was kept confidential. As it is in the confession booth, so it is with the Fed: what banks say is secret. One submission by Citigroup had half its pages obscured by magic marker. An application by Lehman Brothers, 500 pages in length, was all withheld except twenty six pages. It is dangerous, the regulators think, for the public to know too much. But how can the buyer beware when the rules are all secret?

A Fed governor named Gramlich admits there's a problem. The word "scourge" is used, and then quickly qualified. There's a need for study, he says. There's a need for public comment, not against mergers, but on the abstract issue which the Fed puts in quotation marks. "Predatory lending." The banks complain that this term is not defined. But when states propose laws that make the definition crystal clear, the banks lobby against it. It is good to leave it loose, they think. They can say they're against it without changing what they do. When cities pass local ordinances directed at the problem, a concept is invoked that might surprise the Founding Fathers: preemption. When the larger body legislates, the smaller unit can't. Towns in California tried to cap teller fees. The laws were thrown out, at the urging of the Comptroller of the Currency, who "regulates" -- quotation marks are needed -- all national banks. New York has a quaint prohibition on usury, but for naught: any national bank, set up in South Dakota or Delaware, can circumvent it. States pass easy laws to attract lenders' headquarters. There are dozens of banks in Sioux Falls, South Dakota, and an equal fleeing number in Salt Lake City, Utah. It's a race to the bottom: the jurisdiction which regulates least, gets the jobs. Then others weaken their laws to compete. In the U.S. and beyond, it's a jungle.

6.

There are, of course, the freedoms of speech and of the press. The scourge of redlining is annually exposed, using data that's filed pursuant to the Home Mortgage Disclosure Act. The Ur text of this genre was a series in the Atlanta Journal-Constitution called "The Color of Money." It revealed how African Americans were denied loans four times more frequently than similarly-situated whites. A small bank named Decatur was sued, and quickly settled. The larger banks barely changed their practices.

The new buzzword, predatory lending, is becoming a media mainstay. More graphic even than a loan denial is a widow who's slated to lose her home. Sixty Minutes and Primetime Live have hoed this row for television broadcasts. Even the Wall Street Journal has printed, snickering, the most egregious cases. The first protagonist was The Associates, with its high-rate loans for meat. A man in Alabama paid thousands of dollars in interest and fees to buy his pork and chicken in advance. It was a Page One feature, complete with pencil drawing. But when Citi bought this lender, the Journal applauded the business savvy of Sandy Weill, Citi's once and future chairman. He was feted as CEO of the Year; his donations of blood money for the naming-rights to hospital wings was respectfully reported. If profit's the only measure, then the purchase of loan sharks makes sense.

If stock prices are like football or movies, as by the media's focus appears to be the case, then reporters need access to the coaches and moguls. This is how the discipline (not to say censorship) works: the grant or denial of access. The financial press needs face-time with Sandy. If they dig in the gutter and expose Sandy's sins, Citi's scoops will be directed to more compliant outlets. This is a global phenomenon: in Edinburgh the Royal Bank of Scotland demanded a particular journalist be taken off its beat. The ink-stained wretch stood tall, and was then encouraged to resign. This was a story it was not in his interest to tell: he would be blackballed. The carrot of face-time, the advertising stick: but who'll watch the watchers?

7.

There are those who blow the whistle, and they also have their reasons. Prior to CitiFinancial's settlement, three long-time employees had issued sworn statements. There was Gail Kubiniec, who worked in Tonawanda. She said she was trained to forced-sell insurance. There was Michelle Handzel, who corroborated this statement and more. Through a different channel there was a man name Steve Toomey. He cast light on his colleagues, who'd been paid to say nothing. To pay for silence is at least a form of carrot. To fire the whistle blower -- as happened to Kelly Raleigh, *see* Chapterettes 13, 25 and 46 below -- is more akin to a stick. While it could seem illegal, there's a longstanding doctrine called "employment at will." Like debt peonage, the concept is mediaeval. One serves at King Sandy's pleasure. Off with her head!

* * *

It is important to ask how this madness began. Because it's the largest, we'll start with Citigroup. Its beginning, like its end, was as a subprime lender. Sanford Weill, hard-charging Brooklynite on hiatus, bought a bottom-fishing company that was called Commercial Credit. Its headquarters, then as now, was in Baltimore City. It ran hundreds of storefronts in marginal towns. It lent at high rates and it force-placed insurance. It settled some charges with the Federal Trade Commission; it beefed up its network with a purchase from Barclays.

But this wasn't enough, for the hungers of Sandy and the team he had built. There was a lawyer named Prince and a math-whiz named Willumstad. Later a woman named Marge Magner joined the cabal. They wanted more and soon they got it, in the form of the much-sued A.L. Williams insurance company. This they branded as Primerica, a slick mix of patriotism and we're-number-one. This was a more visceral scam: rather than wait in the storefront, Primerica would come to you. Like Amway and other pyramid schemes, it recruited new members and gave them commissions. They in turn found new blood, new victims. They asked you your dream right there in your kitchen, then opened their briefcases with documents to sign. "Sell whole life and invest the difference" was their mantra, and it almost made sense. Except that the investments they offered were second-rate and shoddy.

The trick of Sandy Weill is to cut out the middleman. Why sell others' product when you can brew your own? Or buy a brewery, as the case may be. They bought Travelers Insurance and took on its vaunted name. They bought Smith Barney and left that brand in place. They grabbed Salomon Brothers, then a loan shark franchise called Security Pacific. Driving the onslaught was the profit from storefronts. They developed a system to track their employees. It was mockingly called Maestro: the computer chirped when a sales-chance was missed. "Always be closing," it went without saying. The final trophy Sandy needed was a bank. And soon he would get one.

8.

There was a problem of course -- but it was only a law. Wall Street's crash of 1929 had led to some restrictions. They called it Glass-Steagall. It prevented insurers and securities firms from also controlling a bank. Attempts had been made to break down this wall, but small banks and consumers had in each case fought back. The last years of Clinton were the best window yet. The market was booming and the Dems had gone corporate. Glass-Steagall remained after a '98 onslaught. Then Sandy gave the wall a push.

One Monday in April a bombshell was dropped: Sandy'd buy Citi, all firewalls be damned. The New York Post screamed, "The Deal of the Century." Some asked if it would be illegal. "Only under current law," came the answer. Because laws, like history, belong to the victors.

The range of complaints at the time was quite broad. Commercial Credit had been charged with loan sharking; Salomon Brothers had paid a big fine. Travelers Insurance was said to redline; Smith Barney was arbitrating a slew of sexist scandals, the largest of which was called the Boom Boom Room. At a branch on Long Island, the boys drank Bloody Marys from big garbage cans. Strippers were summoned and then the real meat: the whores. Women who worked there were scoffed at and fondled. When they sued, Sandy's response was mandatory arbitration.

The first of the bankers' injunctions was this: safety and soundness, a strong financial system like plumbing in a house. To give the largest bank to a loan shark like Sandy: was it wise? Alan Greenspan seemed to like it. It would lead to yet more mergers and the Dow Jones average climbed. This was Greenspan's measure; he saw his mug on glossy. The details of an outmoded statute were much less important.

9.

There were, of course, opponents. In high postmodern fashion, this text's originator was among them. From the tabloid Daily News, consider this invective: "'For groups that are focused on banking in poor neighborhoods, this is the one to go to the mat on. This is a watershed,' said Matthew Lee, the activist attorney behind Bronx-based Inner City Press / Community on the Move. 'They need to get fairer, and if they don't get fairer, their application should be denied.'"

The how's-and-why's of location and pedigree are not our concern here. Rather, the context: the Community Reinvestment Act is a law that's on the books. To combat redlining, it requires that banks serve the poorest of neighborhoods. It is enforced on mergers, through comments to regulators opposing the deals. Let's call it ICP -- in Spanish, *La Prensa del Pueblo* -- and jump forward in the action. A hearing is held, at the Fed's castle near Wall Street. Travelers, it seems, is not without defenders. With the money from storefronts, Sandy's bought friends. He's gotten a hospital wing named after himself. He is repairing, and renaming parts of, Carnegie Hall. Sandy's *consigliere* Chuck Prince is in attendance, smirking from his entourage, assured of approval. In this kangaroo court, there's no cross-examination. It's a ritual theater, and not without its costs: "Michael Green, a member of Bronx, N.Y.-based Inner City Press-Community on the Move, had to spend an hour on the subway, miss half of a workday, and bring a Spanish-speaking translator to testify...at the hearing on Citicorp's deal with Travelers Group. But he said the hassle was worthwhile because it gave him the chance to speak out on how his community would be hurt. 'It is very important to come, because maybe they will take it more seriously,' Mr. Green said through a translator."

Among the things lost in translation is the will of the people. The money on the table -- $83 billion -- is simply too much. The merger is approved; the law be damned. What's now called Citigroup is not without a plan. Having broken the law, they will now have it repealed. The Senator in charge is a Texan, name of Gramm. He too knows a chance with he sees it: he will repeal Glass-Steagall if another law goes down. The CRA, Gramm says, is nothing but extortion.

To counter this charge, there's a trade association. The National Community Reinvestment Coalition, it is called, with an office near the White House. There are meetings, there are studies; there is Jesse and then there's the closer. His name is Robert Rubin and he is king of the Wall Street liberals. He ran Goldman Sachs and then, per Time, he ran the universe. He assuages Gramm by reducing the scope of the CRA law. Then he declares victory and takes a job at Citigroup.

10.

Citi, of course, is not alone in this sleaze. More silent but equally deadly is Household Finance. They have bought Beneficial; they make loans against tax refunds at rates of four hundred percent. When challenged, they settle, but always on the cheap. The tax refund cases they manage to dodge: the defendant, they say, is called H&R Block. To clean up their books, they find the right lawyers. In Judge Posner's people's court, in the city of big shoulders, the scam is described:

[T]wo lawyers who had prosecuted two of the unsuccessful class actions, Howard Prossnitz and Francine Schwartz, had lunch in Chicago with Burt Rublin, who was and remains Beneficial's lead lawyer in defending against the class-action avalanche. Prossnitz and Schwartz brought with them to the lunch another lawyer, Daniel Harris. Although neither Prossnitz nor Schwartz, nor their friend Harris, had a pending suit against Beneficial (or against Block, which was not represented at the lunch), they discussed "a global RAL settlement" with Rublin. It is doubtful whether Prossnitz or Schwartz even had a client at this time; and certainly Harris did not. Schwartz later "bought" a client from another lawyer, to whom she promised a $ 100,000 referral fee. The necessity for such a transaction, when the class contains 17 million members, eludes our understanding...

Block was included in the settlement negotiations, despite the fact that there were by then no claims pending against it. It was included because Beneficial was reluctant to settle without Block, having promised to indemnify it for any liability resulting from Block's role in Beneficial's refund anticipation loans. In fact the settlement class received no consideration for the release of any claims against Block. The only effect of bringing Block into the settlement was to allow Beneficial to cut its own expense of the settlement in half. The lawyers for the settlement class were richly rewarded for negotiations that greatly diminished the cost of settlement to Beneficial from the level that it had considered to be in the ballpark years earlier when the cases were running more in its favor than when the settlement agreement was negotiated.... All things considered, we conclude that the district judge abused his discretion in approving the settlement. 288 F.3d 277 (2002)

There are terms of art for this: a reverse auction process to find disarmed counsel. A corporate wrongdoer wants to be sued, to buy atonement on the cheap. They go in search of likeminded lawyers, who will sell out their clients in return for a fee. A class action is filed and then quickly settled. The members of the class get pennies on the dollar but waive all their claims. The lawyers take their fees and the company is henceforth bulletproof. When home loans are at issue, the waiver that's signed is particularly pernicious: when the lender forecloses, there are no defenses. If the loan was made through fraud, it no longer matters. They've paid for that sin and now the loan is clean. It is lucrative for everyone except the consumers.

11.

While this sounds like organized crime, that is not how it's put at the time of recruitment. To get their employees, CitiFinancial and HFC don't say "come and be predatory." Citi says, come get on the train before it leaves the station. You will work for Sandy Weill. He has always doubled money; why should it now be different? The hardest-chargers are given a dream: one day they too can sell stocks, ride jets, wear flashy gold watches like Charles Plumeri. Primerica holds revival-like meetings in Madison Square Garden. It's a form of religion: heaven re-branded as economic freedom. The National Association of Securities Dealers holds the keys to selling stock. It's called the Series 7, or among its initiates, simply The Seven. From loan shark to Wall Street: that is the offer.

There are also incentives to help you along. Citi pays bonuses based on a board game. They call it ROCopoly; its logo is a rotund man in a top hat. You must sell insurance to get Rocco's pay. You must sell more loans, and then collect on them. When there's no money left in your customer's house, you can advance the due-date by several different means. You can make a new loan or get a deferment. The stats are chalked up and the winners rewarded. The cream of the crop is flown to the Islands. Under Carib sun, the loan sharks rest like lizards. Sometimes it's Vegas, sometimes only amusement parks. In the Carolinas, it's Six Flags Over Jesus. There are coffee mugs and hats for those slow to learn. For those with ambition, it's always The Seven. There's a broker at Citi who made thirty million. His name was Jack Grubman and you could be him. Your children, like his, could attend the best schools. There will be no waiting list, not when Sandy can donate a million Citi dollars. As this was being written, Jack Grubman was fired. The change of his rating on AT&T required some neo-Japanese falling on the sword. But he got extra millions to not rat out Sandy. There is only one king in this rat nest: there will be no successor.

12.

After buying a new law, Citi bought a new loan shark. It had been on TV as the worst of the worst: Associates First Capital, headquartered in Senator Gramm's stomping grounds in Texas. That Associates had settled race discrimination charges was a mere inconvenience. While the U.S. victims cried, Citi was two steps ahead. Associates was already in Calcutta, with high-rate loans for what's there called two-wheelers. The British magazine *The Banker* uses the magic word: CitiFinancial Retail "sells consumer loans to underbanked, subprime customers, to buy PCs, durables, and two-wheelers... HSBC has 800,000 customers in India, the second highest in Asia after Hong Kong." These two banks are competing, HSBC and Citi. (The non-bank GE is also in the mix.) Other than in Asia, Citigroup moves first. After Associates, they turned due south to Mexico. Sandy had breakfast with President Fox. The sellers, Banacci Acival, dropped their lawsuits against gadfly reporters. ICP faxed its comments to Mexico City. The U.S. Fed, it was clear, would not give a damn.

Banacci had been bailed out; for a moment some thought that Sandy'd repay the debt. But this is not Sandy's way. After some *cacique* schmoozing, the deal was approved -- but on a condition. The Federal Reserve, unable to rebut evidence of predatory lending, declared that CitiFinancial will be examined at last. The Fed has the staff; it trades in the dollar and lives on the profit. Alan v. Sandy'd be some fight to see. But it's all confidential: ICP deployed the still-standing law, the Freedom of Information Act. The Fed responded with pure legalese, saying it withheld eight linear feet of documents. Like priest and penitent, Alan digests each of Sandy's many sins in silence. It will be the same with Enron. It is not pretty; the security is tight. Snakes, some say, can swallow whole phone booths. But Citi is larger and harder to chew.

13.

Once again there's a problem: the blowing of whistles. In South Carolina there's a man named Steve Toomey. He's a regular bloke, not a saint, nor claiming to be one. But he witnessed hard-selling and forgery too. He writes for ICP his sworn statement:

Until May 24, 2001, I worked as a loan officer at the Charleston, South Carolina, branch of CitiFinancial... It was routine practice to show borrowers the required Real Estate Settlement Procedure Act (RESPA) documents for the first time at loan closings. The RESPA documents were generally not sent out during the required three-day period, but rather were back-dated at the closing.

Before closing loans, we loan officers were required to collect the prospective borrowers' "pay-offs" from other lenders. These "pay-offs" can only be obtained with the written authorization of the prospective borrower. I inquired with a senior employee at my office, and watched as the employee forged the prospective borrower's name on the authorization forms. This happened a number of times.

After Citigroup acquired The Associates, an announcement was made that we loan officers should cease closing loans at borrowers homes. However, the branch executive in charge of the Charleston office (as well as the Columbia and Greenville offices), Tim Delapaz, stated that his supervisor, Steve Diubaldo, told him that we should continue closing loans at borrowers' homes. I am also aware of instances where management falsified commission information and required employees to falsify information in borrowers' files.

I can confirm, and participated in, "Loan Blitz Nights." At my office, these were Tuesday and Thursday evenings (for a time, the days were Monday and Wednesday), and including proposing new loans to existing borrowers, under the compensation scheme described above, which promoted "flipping." The individuals we were to target were identified in a computer system called "Lead-Net."

I declare under penalty of perjury that the foregoing is true and correct.

EXECUTED on July 8, 2001, in Charleston, South Carolina.

Following this filing, Mr. Toomey was not executed. Rather, he was paid a settlement to speak of this no more. Two of his colleagues were not, however, so lucky. They had already signed gag orders, to receive their last paycheck. They spoke to ICP as anonymous sources. Nonetheless they got called by Citi's attorneys. "My name is Mitch," the caller said. "I'm with the firm of Skadden Arps -- I defended Bill Clinton against Paula Jones. And now I want to talk to you." He threatened to sue them if they spoke against Citi. Upon leaving the company they'd agreed to, for life, not disparage The Group. Any damages, Mitch said, they would have to pay. They stopped talking. Alan Greenspan shrugged.

14.

There are more than two sinning banks: we focus here on the large. The bank called Norwest was long subprime-adept. They came to The Bronx with a Latino tinge: Island Finance, they called it. The rates were twenty five percent, the state's usury cap. There was no review of credit histories, just "*Se Habla Español*," this is what you pay. ICP complained, to the weekly Village Voice. In time Norwest closed down its storefront.   Borrowers were required to travel to Queens to keep paying. Then Norwest merged with Wells Fargo, and took their scam up to Alaska.

There is also AIG, the American International Group.   Their roots are in China but their eyes are on the bottom line. They bought American General, a high-rate lender, including on dogs.   They schmoozed their way through every approval; their general counsel, ex-Fedman Ernest Patrikis, threatened to sue ICP. Then he offered to lunch, and then he disappeared. The approvals had been obtained, there was no reason to listen. AIG moved on to strong-arm China. AIG held the keys, via Bush, to the World Trade Organization. They got their special rights. If, as the stereotype has it, they eat dogs in China, why should they not insure them as well?

Small but salacious was the lender named PinnFund. Its chairman was horny; he courted a porn star, while targeting African Americans with his toxic high-cost loans. ICP raised this, on a Japanese bank. When the house of cards tottered, the horndog went south. Later he pleaded guilty, or perhaps *no lo contendere*. The bimbo kept the house -- unlike the borrowers.

In subprime auto lending, there was Mercury Finance: it exploded. In mobile home lending there was Green Tree, which sold itself to Conseco and then wilted. Later GE bought it. *The Money Store* blew up and was re-branded HomEq. NationsCredit was closed; EquiCredit was sold to a 'Net bank. Household bought Decision One. This is called consolidation; it's an unending game. Fly-by-night lenders spring up like mushrooms. Some are taken-out at a substantial premium. Others, like New Century, simply want to be sold.

15.

Some banks like Citi jump deep in with two feet. Others want the profits without the *agita*. U.S. Bancorp, for example, owned a quarter of New Century. When ICP raised it, they sold off their stake. They still serve as trustee; they're still in the game. They are tracked, if at all, through their SEC filings. Since Edgar (dot com) is free, the tracking continues. The balance is profit versus reputational harm. The more obscure the connection, the harder to prove. Goldman, Mizuho, UBS and Paine Webber: through veils of subsidiaries, their ghetto-hooks are hidden.

But take, for example, Credit Suisse and DLJ. When they merged, it was viewed as an investment bank taking over a brokerage. But both were in deep in what they call the subprime space. Credit Suisse underwrote for Green Tree and Conseco; they did it for Delta and Contifinancial. DLJ, like Lehman Brothers, got further down in the gutter. It took a 49 percent stake in Quality Mortgage USA, a California-based lender that was the successor to Guardian Savings & Loan, shuttered by the Resolution Trust Corporation. Both Guardian and its Quality spin-off were run by Russell Jedinak, a king of hard-lending whose slogan was and is, "if the owner has a pulse, we'll give them a loan." (See, *Money of the Mind*).

DLJ Mortgage Acceptance Corporation purchased the Quality loans to securitze them. But these pools of loans were thereafter repeatedly downgraded; through time they became known as the worst performing pools in the history of the mortgage-backed securities market. So DLJ set up Calmco Servicing to handle the loans. A June 30, 2000, SEC filing obliquely stated that Calmco as established as "a subsidiary of the underwriter and an affiliate of the depositor to perform default servicing for approximately 30,000 subprime residential mortgage loans."

Default servicing, also known as collections, is at once photogenic and disgusting. How can water be squeezed from a stone? Used cars can be repo-ed at night; new loans can be made, with other co-signers. Threats, baseball bats -- this is what the journalists make appointments to see. The vast field of screwing is reduced to its final *denouement*: in films of a certain ilk this is called, not without subprime resonance, the "money shot."

16.

If Houdini could escape from a locked steamer trunk, why can't these victims simply re-fi their loans? They could find a lower rate and move their account, no? No. Welcome to the world of pre-payment penalties. Like a prenuptial agreement, to end this abusive marriage requires a lump sum payment. It is set so high that few can afford it. Beyond debt peonage, this is like indentured servitude. The term of the pre-pay might run four or five years. Some have reduced it to two, but it is still indefensible. Some say they waive it if the refi is with a company within their conglomerate. Not so with Household: if one's loan was with HFC's Decision One, the lump sum would still be required. It can, of course, be refinanced. This is a trap more effective than pre-pay: if the loans, taken together, are worth more than the house, no one will refi, no one will help. Loan-to-value ratios of 125 percent are not unknown. They were advertised by the Miami Dolphins' Dan Marino. They are common today at Household Finance.

A variation on the pre-pay game is to simply refuse to accept them. When a customer shows up at CitiFinancial with the offer of a better loan, the pay-off documents are often not given. Employees are told to delay and to talk. Suddenly Citi offers a new and lower rate. "We did you at twelve? We could re-do you at ten." What changed in the interim is never explained. The credit score's no different; only two months have passed. Ten was the baseline that Maestro suggested. The two extra point were just gravy, fodder for bonus or trips to Las Vegas. "We can't find the documents," is often what's said. "But by the way we can now offer ten." As the soul song has it, you better shop around. Because once the hooks are in, they're not easy to get out.

17.

When Household bought Benny, they changed all the rules.
Beneficial Finance paid its workers a salary. With Household the focus
was on the commissions: a percentage on loans. Often the bonus was
company stock. The problems arose when the stock price went down.
The employees of Enron were left with just paper. The HFC gang saw
their retirements decline by two-thirds. So too with Citi, when Sandy's
magic left. For a moment the scam was discussed in the Congress. Then
attention moved on to Iraq War II. Worker beware is the rule of this
jungle. Get the money today since the future's uncertain.

This age, we are told, is a time for free agents. The era of the
Brand-Called-Me. Those with degrees, they can telecommute. We
could *all* be consultants, if someone would pay. Felix Rohatyn, over
frogs' legs, can advise HSBC on its subprime foray. The workers being
bought do not have the same freedom. It's a punch-the-clock world. To
screw the poor you must still have a presence. The storefront, the coffee:
a place, as in a bar, where they all know your name. "Hello, Mrs. Vargas
-- what can we do you for today?"

When government abdicates, there's only the market. With
perfect information, honestly doled, it all still might work. Let
conscience, some say, vote with its feet. If Nike works with sweatshops,
who will buy their sneakers? Millions, it appears, even in the inner city.
The industry forms its own commissions, the companies declare
themselves clean. Why bank with a loan shark? If the face that you see
in the branch is inviting, the distant rumble that something is out there is
not so important. With Citigroup.com, you can pay your bills online. So
what, they screw the poor in China -- let *their* hundred flowers bloom.
What is not represented can be said to not exist. What is the sound of
one loan shark flapping? If a bat falls in a forest and nobody hears, did it
fall?

We count on the media to mirror the world. But the need to sell
ads has now made it a funhouse. The tales of the victims don't stoke our
desires. We would rather see mobsters or faded ex-rockers. If the
victims are richer, it's news you can use. And so the crusades of the New
Democrats. Take Elliot Spitzer, the forehead of Wall Street. The targets
are slick: the big who will settle. Those saved are described as being
small investors. That in truth they fall into the top two percent is the
story's main flaw. But if the poor won't vote why save them? If they

don't donate, they will not have a voice. Those who invest can also contribute. Campaign finance reform, if not total, won't solve this problem.

18.

There arose in the states an outcry about Household. Attorneys general, smelling blood, met *en-masse* in Chicago. The HFC racket is run from a suburb. At length they discussed, then finally a deal. If Household paid half a billion, it could say it was clean. ICP heard from sources that a scandal was known: over twenty thousand victims were simply not counted. But the press releases had already gone out. No time to turn back; the camera lights were on.

Household's CEO is a man named Aldinger. His second is command is Dave Schoenholz. The guy, on a Net-cast, is quite skeletal. He says their business model has withstood the test of time. To stock analysts they claim that to settle was smart. "We resolve the litigation, and for ten cents a share. What we give up in fees can be made back in the rate." The analysts nod and then confirm their ratings. The bond spreads narrow and a sale is drawing near.

HSBC is described as sure-footed. They like to buy assets that are on their last legs. Near-dead banks in Sao Paulo, Brazil; Credit Commerciale de France with its shady Marseillaise; Republic New York with its toxic Russian book. So too with Household: it was bought on the cheap. Its price began Oh-Two at a tad over sixty. By the Fall it had fallen to twenty. To buy at thirty-one was like cheap electronics. Like ol' Crazy Eddy, the prices were *in-saaane*.

Putting the lipstick on a hard-to-catch pig: this Aldinger could do through the use of incentives. A new bonus was offered. Four hundred dollars to re-write bad loans. Those called delinquent, deadbeat for six months, were cold-called and schmoozed. "We can offer a deal if you come to the storefront." New contracts were drawn to conceal the defaults. What Sir John knew, and when he knew it, is not known. He traveled to Scotland and puffed up the deal. To hedge funds in Europe and then to New York. It's called a road show; the host was Morgan Stanley. HFC, it was said, was just misunderstood. It was mostly not subprime! See Aldinger's pie chart, in hues of blue and red. For those who listened closely, the footnotes were there. Any loan secured by real estate they now said was prime. That the rate was high and the payments behind was not now so important. "We serve the mainstream" became Household's cry. Sir John was a knight; creative accounting is Empire's hallmark. It is the house in which Household and Citigroup live.

19.

There are bookworms who feast on the quarterly earnings. They are paid to be skeptics but their voices are drowned out. Bought off with some entrée to elite nursery schools. Fired when bearish; paid to be bulls... One named Tom Brown used to torment First Union. He was fired but reemerged as a telecommuting contrarian. Most are not so lucky, so they just go along. Call it not subprime? Fine. Vote for a merger whose terms are not known? Fine, as long as the spread leads to bonus. Paying those who watch to raise both their thumbs is money well spent. The critics of Household's accounting restatements were missing in action. "Are there gremlins?" was the question. If there were, old Sir John would moonlight as exorcist. At thirty-one dollars, it just didn't matter. Buy now, pay later. The roll call of those arbitraging the deal was not short. By their domain names shall ye know them:

ccorrea@Lehman.com
howard.burdett@abnamro.com
ira.gorsky@us.cibc.com
Jpark@us.nomura.com
jon.guillory@soros.com
yevgeniya.kostareva@db.com (Deutsche Bank)
rstephens@mwe.com (law firm which represented Household)
cffurtado@debevoise.com
DGreen@GibsonDunn.com
ifsam.com (owned by Dutch bank ING)
cdcixis-cmna.com (owned by CDC IXIS)
satellite-ny.com (Satellite Asset Management)
amaranthllc.com
OscarGruss.com
TaconicCap.com
TiedemannFunds.com
wsaccess.com (Wall Street Access)
saghill.com
bear.com (Bear Sterns)

mteichman@ReedSmith.com

This last one bears comment: Michael Teichman was, in 1998, the Delaware Deputy Attorney General who fended off ICP's opposition to Citicorp - Travelers. Four years later, he's paid by Reed Smith to observe ICP's fight against HSBC - Household, at the Delaware Department of Insurance. The bureaucrats angle for subsequent jobs. That the results are corporate-friendly should surprise no one. The banks are so big, they will not be let fail. Their get-out-of-jail-free card is the specter of systemic risk. If Citigroup fails, incumbents will lose. So, Citigroup will not fail. Its cases will settle, and often on the cheap. Even eager Spitzer knows the rules of this game. There's no ticket to Albany, or later-who-knows the White House, as Sandy Weill's slayer. Some blows for the camera; blows of a different kind when the lights go down. Those who are paranoid just might be right.

20.

And so the hair-shirts with their Web sites: Jeremiahs in cyberspace, e-voices in the wilderness. A dozen observers complained about Household. Where, they asked, was the merger agreement? The week of Thanksgiving, ICP wrote it up. It was not Fair Disclosure to play hide-the-ball: this was filed with the SEC and e-mailed to Bloomberg. There was interest but no story ensued. Who were these Bronxites to play in this world? Only AFX, from their Hong Kong newsroom, dared repeat that the Emperor was perhaps without clothes:

In a filing with the SEC, Inner City Press/Community on the Move questioned the completeness of information released to date by the companies concerning the quality of Household International's asset portfolio and a settlement over claims of predatory lending... In the document [ICP] questioned the accuracy of Household's statement that 63 percent of its customer base is "prime" lending... Referring to the company's proposed predatory lending settlement with 19 state attorneys general, [ICP] said in the filing that this Oct 11 in principle "relates solely into home-secured loans." As such, it "does not ... address the issues and risks surrounding the company's high-rate tax refund anticipations loans", whose interest rate he cited legal judgements as attesting "will often exceed 100 pct".

But since the stock price rose, it must not have any merit. That this was Hang Seng's tide was not so important. The elephants were horny. Let the Comstocks be damned. What was wanted from The Bronx was only the victims. "Show us the face of payday lending abuse" -- the Times and News simultaneously asked. The answer was dry and involved Patton Boggs, a lobbying firm throwing blocks for Check n' Go. This is not photogenic; this is not the Bronx' objective job. The Bronx is an object. Like the Zoo it's a place to see but not hear. No victims, no story: it's as simple as that.

That only the printers have the freedom of press is old hat. The internet expands liberty while offering offshore casinos and hidden dorm cameras. The SEC complaint's online; so too some hearsay the mainstream ignores. There are shops that sell dirt to those in the market. *La Prensa* is free: but can it be believed?

21.

There are things lawyers know that they will not reveal. Only as background, with no attribution. For example Montana: two lawyers there know of Citigroup's game. Citi's class action settlement, in the case called *Morales*, is an anti-poor joke. The plaintiffs' attorney will take half of the money. Their clients, for a hundred bucks, will waive all their rights. This is known in Montana but the sources can't be named.

There is a case called *Wombold*, filed in Great Falls, whose file tells the story. The judge is named Macek and here are some facts: "The Wombolds' loan with Citigroup has a principal of $57,000 and another $18,000 in unpaid interest fees on a home Jim Wombold said would sell for $50,000.... They borrowed $9,000 to pay for a dental bill, real estate taxes and some appliances. They used their house at 1521 6th Ave. N.W. as collateral. At the time, they owed $4,000 on the home they bought in 1965... Jim Wombold became disabled in 1997, but the three-year policy expired after just a few payouts. When Elizabeth Wombold broke her ankle the same year and was unable to work, they started to fall behind on the $716 monthly payments owed to Associates. The cost of the expired policy is included in the loan principal... Citigroup spokeswoman

Anita Gupta said her company will not comment on the matter because it is in litigation." Great Falls Tribune, Oct. 2 and 11, 2002. ICP retransmits, gives the numbers of these lawyers to other reporters offline. It will not be reported: the press has moved on. The focus is Sandy and will he survive. The plight of the Wombolds is not worth reporting. It's always this way, before the Great Falls. Anyway, the lawyers who propose now to settle with Citi are racking up fees: $375 an hour for "extensive Internet research;" the same fee for travel. Later, Citigroup will defend this payola. Anything to get a waiver and put the past behind them.

22.

For the titans of Wall Street like Sandy, the media is mostly a boudoir mirror: it shows what they want it to. By controlling access and face-time, the reporters let into the fold are pre-screened. The gatekeeper at Citi is one Leah Johnson. She is as loyal as a pit bull. Her allegiances have shifted over the years. In 1991 she flacked for the NYC Districting Commission. Then a stint in politics with Hevesi, then the S&P, McGraw Hill and finally Citi. She would fall on her sword for Sir Sandy. The feeling's not mutual.

Sandy's connections go much further back. There's a woman at Fortune, for example, who can always be counted on to save Sandy's bacon. As the SEC closes in, as Spitzer leaks to the Journal's Charles Gasparino, there's always this outlet, as much space as Sandy needs. The woman's not even a journalist: she moonlights, more lucratively, editing the annual reports for Warren Buffet's Berkshire Hathaway. Still she gets exclusive quotes, and the other journos pine. Sandy at Rest. Sandy Fights Back.

Sandy is angry at Charles Gasparino. The reasons are personal: when Sandy's son Marc fell asleep at his desk, with burn-marks on his fingers that all knew were crack, Gasparino wrote it up. In this now-blurry timeframe, Marc Weill bought a stake in the subprime lender IMC. It teetered near failure then Citi stepped in. There were losses, yes. And reputational hits which, unlike Associates, Sandy'd not chosen. Marc went to rehab, then hid in the phone tree. He works somewhere in Citigroup, no one's sure where. Sandy's daughter started her own brokerage, whose Initial Public Offering her proud papa couldn't even underwrite due to conflict of interest. To attack a man's family is going too far. Even if, through nepotism, they buy subprime lenders.

Leah for Sandy has attacked ICP. When the Carolina gag orders were being reported by Reuters, Leah sent a statement rebutting this narrator by name. "She *really* doesn't like you," two journos reported. This feeling's not mutual: she's just doing her job. Where in The Hague that defense is accept is still not clear.

23.

Beyond compliant press, one can always name buildings. The guru of Tyco, for example, has a monument at Seton Hall College. Ken Lay of Enron has business school lecture halls named after him. There are moves afoot to bury this history, but a contract's a contract. "It will make them think of ethics," one dean was heard to say. For a brief moment this archaic word was in the news: ethics. Then the calls for war and the mid-term elections. It was only a blip, just a few bad apples, we were told. Those who question America too much have no future.

Clean elections are a buzzword too, but it's largely misleading. Issue ads, the use of planes: there remain ways to buy favors, and Citi plays the game. They got Leon Panetta and even Joe Lockhart. They got Stanley Fischer from the IMF. Household shot lower. They got the Pennsylvania Secretary of Banks, James B. Kauffman. The ex-governor of Washington state, and a single ex-Senator, Connie Mack. This is quickly followed with a used-up, redistricted Dem, John LaFalce. Sir Bond from Shanghai mistook Mack for Orrin Hatch. ICP raised the issue and Business Week backed down: they'd mis*heard* Sir John Bond and would run a correction. Like these luke-warm clean elections, it was only a footnote. So too, for now, Household's over-limit contributions to New York State pols, and its pay-offs to Delaware Insurance Commissioner Donna Lee Williams. This may be important -- but if so, only later. The new Mike Teichman, a Mike named Rich (said, Risch), new counsel to Ms. Donna Lee, admits that money changed hands: from Household to Donna, while Household owned a Delaware insurer. "It strains credulity," he writes, to argue that Household's donation now requires "a recusal in the absence of specific evidence of bias." But that too is coming.

24.

The power of entrée should not be underestimated. It's who you know (or can buy a connection to), not *what* you know. Dinners and junkets both play their roles. The billionaire mayor of the City of New York took Sheldon Silver down for golf in Bermuda. Suntanned and punch-drunk, they struck a budget deal. Later, the terminal king will gain a stay without opposition of the Council's lending law. "The law took effect Feb. 17, [2003] but was stayed by the judge's order. If the law was in effect, it could have prevented any of the underwriters with bank affiliations that could not certify their compliance with the law from doing work for the city. The law required banks to certify that they had not engaged in mortgage lending that the lawmakers said was abusive of borrowers." Citigroup, it seems, had refused to certify. Citi rather flies its private banking clients to dine with Europe's opinion makers. Now-desperate Chase, with its new name J.P. Morgan, does much the same thing. You can join the club with money. Seven course meals have a tendency to soften the edges.

Of Morgan Chase it must be said: they are also in subprime. Chase Manhattan Funding, in some New Jersey suburb, has funded mobile homes. Then on the cheap and without application, Chase bought Advanta. They did subprime cards and home equity loans. Through Texas-based AmeriCredit, Chase will lend on subprime cars. Investment banking is a volatile business. On the other hand the poor you will always have with you. Chase's old statesman, Dave Rockefeller, can get blown by Barbara at will. Baba Wawa, the secret squeeze of Henry the K (Kissinger, not Kravis), will wait endless hours at his Westchester redoubt. He says the "Shah of Iran, on balance, was good. Sure, he tortured some people. But are the Ayatollahs better?" But who *is* Rockefeller, to rule Tehran or even Valhalla? The press puffs his book, memoirs of a tired white man. Charlie Rose is honored to move in these circles. Bloomberg's in the mix, there with the maitre d', paying the bill. He who pays, rules. Even Baba Charlie knows this.

25.

Lower down the food chain there's the Knoxville Ruby Tuesdays. Here there's a showdown, between long-time branch manager Ms. Kelly Raleigh and her Regional Manager. He wants to know: who's been leaking Citi docs to that dirty ICP? Kelly doesn't know, but if she did, she wouldn't say. "Save yourself," she's advised. It's employment at will, in Tennessee and elsewhere. After she's hired, Inner City Press runs her story:

Kelly Raleigh went to work for Commercial Credit in 1990. Through her twelve year career, she would work at and, later, manage, a half-dozen different offices of Commercial Credit then the renamed CitiFinancial. As she was promoted from loan officer to branch manager, she began to see more and more irregularities. She was trained to close loans while covering the actual loan documents with her forearm, so the customer couldn't read them. She declined to do this, choosing instead to describe to the customer the terms of the loan.

Even when the company was named Commercial Credit, it required "property lists" of household items to purportedly secure consumer loans averaging $5,000 to $7,000. Employees were directed to sell insurance on these household items. Ms. Raleigh describes a loan to an elderly woman that was "secured" by a ladder, on which insurance was sold. Routinely, personal property insurance was sold to customers who already had comprehensive homeowner's insurance: a process known as "double-dipping" in which the second insurance policy has no benefit to the customer. Ms. Raleigh states that CitiFinancial employees routinely doctored insurance applications for customers to make them eligible for insurance (selling unemployment insurance to housewives, and changing the ages and medical history of customers). The reason? To get bonuses, employees had to hit ever-rising insurance sales "penetration levels."

Ms. Raleigh's troubles began when she became aware that CitiFinancial was illegally collecting on a loan, and had been for a number of years. The loan was a second mortgage made by the Morristown, Tennessee office. When the borrower died, CitiFinancial did not go to court and obtain a judgment. Rather, it began collecting from the deceased borrower's son. They pressured the son to put up his car as collateral. When Ms. Raleigh became aware of the illegal collection practices, she raised the issue up through the chain of command: to her district manager, to her regional manager, and then even higher. But nothing was ever done. The Morristown branch manager wrote a memo claiming that the borrower was still alive. Ms. Raleigh was instructed to "quit being a cry-baby and just do it" -- that is, collect on it. By then the loan had been transferred from the Morristown office to the Jefferson City office, where Ms. Raleigh was branch manager and therefore again in charge of continuing to collect on the loan. She refused to collect, and advised the deceased borrower's son to seek a refund. She told her supervisors she had given this advice -- "since I have to live with myself," she told them.

When in February 2002 ICP began to report in detail on systemic predatory lending by CitiFinancial, including documentation from branches in Tennessee, Ms. Raleigh and others were summoned to a meeting in the CitiFinancial office in Kingston Pike. The date was April 4, 2002: Ms. Raleigh was told to go to Kingston Pike and to not tell anyone she was going there. Inside, a CitiFinancial auditor from Baltimore was waiting, along with CitiFinancial's outside counsel. Ms. Raleigh was told that this was a deposition; she was questioned about any knowledge she had of documents being "leaked" from CitiFinancial offices. Ms. Raleigh said she had no knowledge. The following day, they visited her at the Jefferson City office, asking pointedly if she had anything else to say. She didn't.

On June 3, 2002, ICP submitted to the regulators documentation of CitiFinancial insurance sold on fishing rods and ice chests, and various internal CitiFinancial memoranda and sales training scripts. On June 25, 2002, Ms. Raleigh was summoned to the CitiFinancial's Broadway office, where she met with CitiFinancial's Director of Investigations and Corporate Security. At this meeting, Ms. Raleigh described at length the consumer protection compliance violations she had witnessed, including illegal collections from a dead man's son, forgery by employees on insurance documents, and systemic distortion of delinquency. To obtain bonuses, reported delinquencies can only be so high. But the numbers can be distorted by, for example, canceling insurance policies so that insurance premium can be reallocated to loan payments. Ms. Raleigh also corroborated

ICP's earlier account of distortion of delinquency: the invocation of "blizzard deferments" on loans when no snow had, in fact, fallen.

"I think you're mis-remembering things," it was repeatedly insisted.

"So I guess you're going to fire me," Ms. Raleigh finally said.

"No," said CitiFinancial's Investigations Director. "You can't be fired for saying this. We're here to get the facts and get this thing fixed."

But it soon became clear to Ms. Raleigh that the "thing" that CitiFinancial wanted to "get fixed" was the leaking of documents reflecting CitiFinancial's practices, and not the practices themselves. On June 26, 2002, the day after the meeting at the Broadway office, Ms. Raleigh was confronted in the Jefferson City office and asked again: who is leaking? Who is keeping diaries of our practices? By now Ms. Raleigh had contacted an attorney; they told them she was represented by counsel, and not to attempt to question her anymore.

But on July 3, both her regional and district managers came to the Jefferson City office and told her she was suspended. When she asked why, she was not given a reason.

26.

Immediately following CitiFinancial's July 3, 2002, suspension of Ms. Raleigh, CitiFinancial changed the locks on her office in Jefferson City, and at the Morristown office as well. Morristown employees were interviewed over two days, and the district manager was observed removing documents from the Morristown to Jefferson City office, where she was observed shredding the documents. Only then was an audit of the Morristown office performed: an audit that the Morristown office not surprisingly passed. What might these shredded documents have reflected? It has been suggested to ICP that they consisted of the paper trail of various fraudulent loans: transactions in which, to sell insurance, customers' ages were changed (so that the age on the ID documents and the applications forms were different); documents concerning loans that CitiFinancial had been illegally collecting on, as so forth.

On July 15, 2002, Ms. Raleigh went to a Ruby Tuesday's restaurant to meet with her regional manager When she got there, he announced that he was waiting for one more person. When this person arrived, it was a female attorney. "But I'm represented by a lawyer," Ms. Raleigh said again. "You can't have a lawyer question me without my own lawyer here." But the questioning proceeded. Ms. Raleigh was asked to provide the names of the people leaking information or she would be prosecuted.

"For *what*?" she asked. When the question wasn't answered, she called her lawyer, who told her to leave Ruby Tuesday's immediately. She did.

On August 13, 2002, Kelly Raleigh received a letter of termination, dated August 7, 2002, and labeled "Overnight Delivery." The letter tersely stated that the cause was her refusal to cooperate with Company management regarding a violation of company policy. The "Company Policy" referred to must be a policy against whistle-blowing: because Ms. Raleigh *repeatedly* sought to report and cooperate regarding exposing and acting on violations of consumer protection policies and laws.

Citigroup then argued that Ms. Raleigh was not a whistleblower under Tennessee law, and claimed that Ms. Raleigh either never brought up consumer protection violations, or that these were not the reason she was suspended and terminated.

In a *he said - she said* situation, when the "he" represents the largest bank in the country and the "she" is a single mother who, among other things, remains a fan of the Cleveland Browns football team, it's not much in question who will win. At least in the short term. ICP raised these issues directly to the Federal Reserve Board and Citi's other regulators. In October 2002, the Fed sent three lawyers down to Knoxville to depose Ms. Raleigh and others. As of this writing, nothing's been done. At the end of October 2002, the Fed curtly said that its examination is ongoing.

27.

To those who track stocks, the truth's not important. What matter is the *perception* of truth, and what those with power will do about it. In the months before the Fall, there was talk of a "Sandy premium." How much higher should Citi's stock trade since Sandy was in charge? And if Spitzer or a bus took him out, how far would the price fall?

With Household there was no management premium. It traded at sixty at the beginning of the year; by late 2002, it was languishing near twenty. A boutique-firm analyst named William H. Ryan said the books were being cooked, the loans being "re-aged." Did Connie Mack put out a hit? No. Rather, they ran to Sir Bond's HSBC. They'd met in a lawsuit -- the possible confusion between HFC and HSBC -- and now they did business. On Oct. 24 Household sold some new stock. Nine hundred million dollars' worth, straight through Goldman Sachs. The price was twenty-one. No disclosure was made, of material discussions to sell off the company, to HSBC or to anyone else. Three weeks later, the deal was done at thirty-one. The Goldman insiders had made a quick killing. But what did the timing mean?

The options were two, and neither was pretty. Either Household had lied, in not disclosing its merger talks with Bond. Or there were no talks when the stock was sold: meaning that HSBC's check-up on Household was done in two weeks. The word in the market is gremlins: would some gremlins emerge, from Household's murky books, letting HSBC walk? Or like they did in Republic, when a scandal hit the news, would the deal-price simply fall? To those who watch stocks, it did not really matter. The perception of untouchability was enough to close the spread, if not necessarily to close the deal.

28.

That nineteen state A.G.'s chose to close the books on Household should perhaps not surprise. It was October 2002, three weeks before elections. To announce a win, and for half a billion dollars, was propitious at that time. And not just the money: the injunctive relief. Household's pre-payment penalties would be reduced from three years to two. Aldinger like Atlas shrugged. He could make up the difference by raising the rates. And, his Web site crowed, it only covered real estate.

On the signature loans, there was no oversight. Nor on the tax loans, the live checks they mail out to lure in new customers, the auto insurance and car-title loans, the sales finance contacts and subprime credit cards. It was a good time for subprime. It was a win-win situation.

Then Sir John swept in, but the deal stayed the same. Why not expand it? ICP asked, in late-night faxed to over 40 states. The return-fire consisted of identical letters from various AGs; only later would the Freedom of Information Act yield the behind-the scenes e-mailing, for ten cents a page. As recited by Sandra Kane of the Arizona AG's Office, "the negotiating team had a conference call yesterday to discuss the letter that Inner City Press has sent to several attorneys general in opposition to the Multi-state settlement with Household and the HSBC acquisition of Household. Attached is a proposed response that the attorney general offices may wish to use." The drafter was David Huey of the Washington State AG's Office; Kathleen Keest of Iowa e-told him, "Superb letter, Dave!" To which he responded: "I bet you say that to all the boys," followed by emoticon.

ICP is no hair-shirt, though this quirky phrase it relies on too much. The idea behind the phrase is self-denial: the wearing of itchy fur inside one's own shirt. ICP for a time cut win-win deals with banks. It began in '92 with the Bank of New York. But in '94 five more deal were struck. Mergers were challenged; discussion were held. HSBC was among them: its Buffalo honchos Pete Davidson and Martin Leibman met with ICP on Wall Street. Their law firm, Cadwalader, had hired the former state Superintendent of Banks. His name is Derrick Cephas and he smiled shrewdly; his pencils were sharp. He drafted agreements replete with Wherefore's. ICP would drop its protest if HSBC would lend fifteen million in the South Bronx and Harlem, and open an office on 148th Street. HSBC did this, after three nights of talks. They put out a press release and then they moved on.

29.

During a challenge to NatWest, for a merger in Jersey, Cephas in limo came up to The Bronx. NatWest's Number Three was along for the ride. His name was Roger Goldman. He was plump and self-assured; he cut right to the chase.

"We'd like to work with your group," he said. "Derrick's told me some of what you do. We've partnered with community groups before, giving grants and whatnot. So talk to me." He stopped and waited. It was an offer to buy ICP out. Cephas leaned forward. "The point of the Community Reinvestment Act is getting *real* money in the hands of *real* people," he said.

Roger Goldman looked angry. "This is not a game," he said. "It's a five hundred million dollar merger. We've promised cost-savings, we've got a time-line. If I were you I'd make a proposal."

"How about a new branch in the South Bronx?"

Goldman laughed, then stopped. Cephas whispered in his ear. "Well I don't know," Goldman finally said. "We're a bank that's growing, as you can see. But the South Bronx? I'm not sure the area could support a branch."

"Since there's so few bank branches, people save their money in cash. Under their mattresses. If you open a branch you'll have customers waiting."

"The South Bronx is a moonscape," Goldman said. "It's like Dresden or something. I've been through it, I've seen it."

"When?"

Goldman rubbed his plump chin. "Maybe six, seven years ago."

"Well it's changed since then." Somewhat.

"Tell you what," Cephas said, "Roger and I are going to drive around this afternoon. Meanwhile, you think about what else you might want, if anything. Here's how the deal would go -- we do a joint press release, you withdraw your protest and agree in writing not to comment on NatWest's mergers in the future."

"And NatWest does what, exactly?"

"It opens a branch," Cephas said, leading Goldman to the door.

Goldman turned back. "You didn't tell us about yourself," he said.

"Maybe another time."

30.

NatWest opened its branch, not far from the courthouse. The other side of ICP was there as a defendant. Its members had fixed a vacant building, but now a developer named Silverstein wanted it. They'd borrowed the power of eminent domain. It was a government project, to spent $100,000 per apartment. The Silversteins' Sparrow Construction took most of it. They sent guys in gold chains to the building at midnight. "You all should really leave," they said. "The Silversteins usually get what they want." The offer was five hundred dollars. Could they return to their apartments? No: the building'd be given to Banana Kelly, a cute name for a now-corrupt group. The offer was rejected and the court cases flew. The eviction papers were signed by Paul Crotty, a previous city housing commissioner now in private practice. But the great man's petition of eviction was sloppy. The case was dismissed and another one started. In eminent domain: there should be compensation. But not to mere squatters, was Paul Crotty's argument. Our response papers cited to the Cross Bronx Expressway. Sixty thousand families lost their homes for that gridlocked public use. Like them, the homesteaders are rudely displaced: a January morning with riot police. A promise to legalize other homesteading buildings is made -- but only if the banks will help. Which they will only do in exchange for silence. This text, one hopes, speaks for itself.

Part II

31.

To speak through the blizzard of voices of victims -- sometimes the only responses are bitter. At four in the morning on November 14th, an e-mail arrives in The Bronx. It's from London, from a then-coffee-drinking ink-stained young wretch. From Columbia J School she got a job at Reuters, then summoned to the city of Blake. This morning she has witnessed a dark Satanic merger announcement: Sir John Bond's HSBC wants to go predatory, buying Household for a song. The e-mail she send to The Bronx she believe will sit in an in-box for hours.

But the Inner City Press never sleeps, at least not while it's dark. Its Fair Finance Watch, stretched as on a wheel over the many sundry time zones, leaps into action. A press release goes out, a single page that asks: has Sir John goes made? The sun is rising in The Bronx when the rolling gate comes down. By afternoon it's on A.P., it's in the Financial Times and even the Wall Street Journal. The imagery is midieaval: a "consumer advocate already has issued a warning to Sir John. Matthew Lee, executive director of Inner City Press/Community on the Move and the Fair Finance Watch, a consumer organization based in the Bronx, N.Y., said the group intends to protest the deal." There's a rattling of sword or sabers; we will suit up in armor, grab a Quixotic lance and charge forward.

Not the why but the where is an ever-moving target. The Hongkong & Shanghai Banking Corporation, founded on the opium trade, is wily and inscrutable. Will they apply to the Federal Reserve? At first it seems yes; then they make an amendment and claim the answer's no. Household owns a savings bank, quaintly called a thrift. But they are dismembering it. They throw a piece to Lehman Brothers, and the nights of the round cluttered table can do nothing. They offer an Oregon piece to an Idaho bank with the aw-shucks name of Panhandle. War-cries fly in the Spokane Spokesman-Review. It is a marginal side-show: an arb from Bear Stearns says so. But to be a Fair Finance Watcher one must be wily, too. One must accept slander; if by e-mail, delete it. As a sample, there's this, from one <fferraro@bendcable.com>:

YOU COULDN'T STOP HSBC FROM TAKING OVER HOUSEHOLD ANY MORE THAN THE MAN IN THE MOON. FURTHERMORE, I

DON'T KNOW OF ANYONE TWISTING ANYONE'S ARM OR PUTTING A GUN TO SOMEONE'S HEAD TO GET THEM TO BORROW FROM HOUSEHOLD. IF SOMEONE DOES NOT LIKE THE TERMS HOUSEHOLD OFFERS-WELL, IDIOT, JUST GO SOMEWHERE ELSE.

Or this, from <bdesrochers@comcast.net>:

Well I hate to say it but that little filing shows what you know about the company I work for and our Rates. That filing will get you nowhere because it shows a total disregard for any research at all on your part, throwing wild accusations about things you clearly don't know anything about. I guess it is only right to keep banging the drum about a company even though it is not true or accurite [sic] any longer. Because a company is willing to take a higher risk on a loan for low to moderate income families to get the money they need you want a 7 percent rate??? If you had any idea how the industry functions you would not be crying fowl [sic] over a higher rate, these people can not go to a bank, if they could they would not be doing business with us! Like the stock market my friend Greater Risk for a Greater Return....it's the laws on Capitalism and a great system it is, but I'm sure you don't know anything about that!

32.

There are, of course, other views. On message boards run by Yahoo! and AOL, Household shareholders and employees kvetch about trading in their stock for the "American Depository Receipts" of this scarcely-known HSBC. "It's the third largest bank in the world, idiot," one opines. The subtext, on the board, is: bunch of Chinks. If only they knew -- the board of directors of HSBC is full of knight, Lords and even a Baroness. Beyond Sir John, there's Sir Brian, he of Corus steel; there's the Antiguan Sir Mark Moody-Stewart, fresh from Shell and now in mining. There's The Lord Butler, and another Lord named Marshall. This last pals around with The Baroness Dunn, who was chased from the board of Marconi due to conflict of interest. There's also a man named David Eldon who's the chairman for Asia for HSBC. It's Eldon who responds, on November 20 to a Reuters reporter in Hong Kong:

HSBC said on Wednesday it hoped a challenge by a U.S. consumer advocate group would not delay its takeover of finance firm

Household International The advocate group, Inner City Press/Community on the Move, has challenged the deal because of what it calls Household's predatory lending tactics.

"I certainly hope it won't delay the deal," said David Eldon, a director of London-based HSBC Holdings. "I think one has come to expect that in any potential takeover there will always be people who will object to certain things whether they are accurate in their objections or not," he told reporters on the sidelines of a business conference. "I certainly would not believe that we have ever done business anywhere that would be consider unethical. It's not our style, not our nature and anybody who know us would have agreed to that."

That same day, the Spanish Commission on the Prevention of Money Laundering and Monetary Infractions imposes a fine of 2.1 million euros on HSBC for money laundering though numbered overseas accounts linked to collapsed brokerage Gescartera.   From Reuters: "925,000 euros for failing to identify account-holders by name, and a further 300,000 euros for not investigating the unusual operation. [Also,] Spain fined the bank 865,000 euros for failing to establish appropriate internal checks to prevent the occurrence."

This is a pattern at HSBC: the Los Angeles Times ("Response to Terror: Money Trail Leads to Gulf Accounts," Oct. 20, 2001) has reported that 9/11 hijacker Marwan "Al-Shehhi, a native of the Emirates, had an account at a local branch of London-based HSBC Holdings." The London Guardian ("Looted $1 billion Sent Through London," Oct. 4, 2001) has reported on the funneling through HSBC of money stolen by Nigeria's ex-dictator Sani Abacha. The Independent (London) of Feb. 22, 2002, reported that HSBC "is co-financing Alstom in its production of turbines for the Yangtze dam, a project that will inflict appalling ecological damage on one of the rivers the money is meant to be targeting."

So there are rivers of money -- from dictators, from terrorists, from authoritarian states intent on displacing millions of their citizens -- and at the center of it all is HSBC. There was only one weapon that their arsenal lacked: a predatory lender. And now they're buying one for less than two times book-value. The markets love it, at least initially. The battle is uphill.

33.

So too for Citi: it emerges that Sandy paid a million dollars, straight from the corporate slush-fund, to get Jack Grubman's kids into nursery school at the 92nd Street Y. It's a New York story, Wall Street buying the Upper East Side in exchange for stock rating upgrades. Eliot Spitzer -- his doppelganger's Swanker -- issues subpoenas for peanut butter and jelly sandwiches without crust. Grubman is jettisoned, with a parachute gold enough to glitter forever. He's been thrown overboard, but with a high-life preserver. Perhaps Sandy will follow. Enron's chief, and WorldCom's too, are faced with prison time. The bald man from Tyco is boating off-shore. Sandy remains, fiddling in his faux-fireplaced office on Park Avenue, ready for all comers. Sandy's arrived where HSBC wants to get. Their transport is by means of a flurry of car repossessions.

To repo is an art form. A man from Rent-A-Center explains: you have to threaten to take even more. While you plug the TV and the VCR, cast glances at the fridge and couch. Even the bed, if they borrowed for that. Surprising, the apathy, except on holidays. The man from RAC has a joke about racking: the back of the TV is in winter full of roaches. Why? "Because it's the warmest place in the house."

These are the punch-lines that they tell at their Vegas retreats. CitiFinancial, for example, brings its top-selling employees down to Puerto Rico each February. It is an honor the like of which Jack Bender can only dream. It is the pot of Cuervo gold at the end of Nancy Peel's rainbow. One day, perhaps, she can live like Zoe Baird, and hire undocumented immigrants to care for her children. Except she'll be too old by then. Nancy is childless. The world is not fair.

34.

What was strong in mid-October is by late November weak. The restitution as the AGs called it was to average $1,500 to Household's victims for the last three years. Some had lost their homes; others' losses ran to high-five figures. "Why didn't you seek enough money from Household to fully compensate all harmed consumers?" It's a frequently asked question, to which the Washington attorney general's web site answered:

> "Our main concern was to provide as much compensation to consumers as possible. Analysts told us that the amount of money Household will be forced to pay still leaves the company financially stable so that they could actually comply with the settlement rather than become insolvent. If we had demanded too much, the company's financial stability could have been put at risk, which could have resulted in no consumer restitution whatsoever." (*See*, www.wa.gov/ago/householdfinance/faq.htm, as of July 4, 2003.)

Perhaps less-frequently asked, this raises other questions. For example, *whose* analysts told the attorneys general that $484 million was all Household could afford to pay? And if HSBC, the third largest bank in the world, now wants to buy Household, doesn't that change the analysis?

In a frenzy in early December, Inner City Press writes to forty AGs, asking just that. It is highly impolitic, questioning these paragons of consumer advocacy. Spitzer, for example -- who can question his motives? (Bender, comes the fictive refrain). A staffer for the Iowa AG is angry: she demands a conference call with ICP. Okay then, let's do it. A staffer from Washington is on the line as well. "You're pushing it too far," the Iowan says. "You're free to oppose HSBC's applications. But to urge a delay in the payments, I just don't understand."

But those who are homeless, will fast low payment help them more than something larger with delay? "Have you even *asked* HSBC?" To that, there is no answer. The settlements are finalized on December 16; from Des Moines there comes a press release. By week's end, Household files its proxy, and the answer is in it. The merger with HSBC is contingent on the settlement not being "materially expanded." For a month there was leverage, but now the leverage is gone.

35.

From A.P. in Des Moines comes some news that's not true: the settlement's unprecedented, and the merger is already done. What? The watching of finance must include fact-checking the media. The A.P. editor in New York is called; he adds a line about "pending regulatory approval." An angry letter is faxed to Des Moines, and the reporters responds. "The attorney general's spokesman told me that," she says. She adds ICP to her story, says she's get the AG later. But the damage is done. The earlier version appears in the dailies. The deal, it's implied, is over and done with. Now the AGs answer, in a flurry of identical letters on heavy-bond stationary from Richmond, Virginia and Harrisburg, Pennsylvania. "You've raised important questions," they say, "that are best address in the state and federal regulatory proceedings concerning HSBC's applications." Okay then. The battles move on.

Meanwhile there's more Citi action. The American Banker runs a piece about Morales, the private class action that Citi is settling. It's in exchange for a waiver of claims, which the Federal Trade Commission couldn't give. Still the FTC supports the lawyers in *Morales*, who stand to make twenty to twenty-five million dollars while gaining only that amount for their clients. The Banker reports that "some complain that consumers are getting far less compared to what they are giving up in their future rights to sue Citi," and that "some critics have questioned, for example, the size of the California plaintiffs' attorney fees." An error in the story is attributable to the FTC: "The largest part of the settlement will go to two million Associates customers who had bought credit insurance. Each will get about $1,000, more than half of the premiums they paid on that insurance, the FTC's Mr. Winston said."

Unlike with the wider A.P., this is an error that can still be corrected. Letters to the editor have a long tradition among kooks:

> In Laura Mandaro's otherwise-illuminating Dec. 13 article ("Citi Moving Fast to Put Associates Suits to Rest"), there is a statement by the Federal Trade Commission's spokesman Joel Winston which doesn't add up, regarding the "two million Associates customers who had bought credit insurance" -- that "Each will get about $1,000, more than half of the premiums they paid on that insurance, the FTC's Mr. Winston said." But if the two million people the FTC is claming to help each got $1000, that would be a $2 billion settlement, eight times more than what the FTC actually settled for.

> We have observed the FTC trying to make its settlement with Citigroup appear to be more meaningful than it is. In fact, it comes to less than $200 per victim, in exchange for them signing a broad release that would prohibit them from raising fraud in the loan-

making even in a foreclosure case against them.   From our perspective, the FTC showed a lack of will in settling on these terms with Citigroup. For example, the FTC's Mr. Winston was previously quoted, in the Buffalo News of Nov. 8, 2001, that the FTC would expand its case beyond Associates to CitiFinancial itself (which never happened). But for the FTC to mislead the public, and your newspaper's readers, about the settlement is going too far. Please correct the FTC's statement, or ask the FTC for a clarification.

The letter quickly runs; the FTC's clarification, like the response to ICP's FOIA request to the FTC, does not come so quickly.

36.

Predatory lending has become a hot topic, or at least a luke-warm one, in the holiday season. A pushy guy from the New York Times calls about payday lending. What is this County Bank in Delaware, he wants to know -- how is it they're permitted to charge 400 percent interest in New York, where the highest rate under law is supposed to be twenty-five? The answer is pre-emption: County is a national bank, and the federal regulators do not have a usury cap. New York law just doesn't apply.

"Interesting," the Timesman comments. But what he wants from the storefront are victims: graphic victim who have clean hands. He's left holes in his story into which he'll fit them. Where are they, he demands -- if this is a scourge, where are the people who's oxen have been gored?

Bad facts about Household are flooding the storefront; attempts are made to direct them to regulators, in the form of case studies. For example: a loan by Household Mortgage Services, Inc. in Knoxville, Tennessee, to an elderly couple. The husband was born in 1922 and is 80 years old; the wife was both in 1931 and is 71 years old. There are two inter-related Household loans: a first mortgage for $103,000 at a 13.5% interest rate, and a related second mortgage for $25,000 at a 14% interest rate. Knox County, Tennessee, has appraised the couple's home to be worth $101,100. The combined mortgage, of $128,000, is at a 127% loan-to-value. The couple is trapped in the loan because it cannot be   refinanced.

There's more: the 71 year old wife works forty hours a week at a

Senior Citizens Center in Knoxville, for $7.01 an hour. Monthly from this job, pre-tax, she earns $1213.33, plus $700 monthly from Social Security. The husband, at 80, can no longer work; his monthly Social Security is $1,084 and he receives a pension benefit, from previous work, of $333 per month. Thus their combined pre-tax monthly income, with the 71 year old wife working, is $3,330.33.

The monthly payment due on Household's first mortgage is $1,091; the monthly payment due on Household's second mortgage is $313, for a total monthly debt to Household of $1,404. That is 42.2% of the couple's total pre-tax monthly income, even before one considers for example the $1,430.57 annual taxes on the house and the couple's other debts, which include semi-secured and auto-secured subprime loans with Citigroup's subprime unit, CitiFinancial.

The "reforms" in Household's settlement with state attorneys general would not prevent this type of loan from being made in the future. The reforms are limited to Household's branch originated business, while these types of loans are made through Household's so-called "correspondent" channel -- that is, through brokers.

Documentation of this loan was sent to HSBC's directors, in Hong Kong, Canada and London. Another example: a Household loan that began on or about May 27, 1997. It began as a second mortgage loan; it began with the forgery of the required proof of employment proof of income. The branch manager of the HFC office signed a Request for Verification of Employment form, with the name of non-existent employer.

Through this fraudulent second mortgage, and as stated in a subsequently filed complaint, Household "repeatedly and persistently telephoned" the borrowers, engaging in "high pressure sale tactics" to induce the borrowers to refinance for more money and at a higher rate. This was done on March 2, 1999, at a fixed interest rate of 16.759 percent. Credit life insurance and credit disability insurance were included "as a term and condition of the March 1999 loan," in an amount far greater than the purported restitution offered through Household's recent settlement of charges of predatory real estate lending."

In response, the borrowers endeavored to contact Household's management, including current CEO William Aldinger. The borrowers then received a telephone call from Aldinger's secretary stating that if the borrowers again attempted to call Aldinger, Aldinger and / or Household would have them arrested.

Since Household's settlement was limited to the complaints the attorneys general had in their files -- this was heard from Iowa, New York Rhode Island and elsewhere -- it should be emphasized that Household has systemically discouraged complaints, including, in this case, by threatening complaining borrowers with arrest.

37.

Unlike old-time loan sharks, the new ones can securitize their debt. They put the loans in a pool and sell the pool in slices (picture black lines against a light blue background under crystalline water). Household has funded its whole business this way. They sell corporate bonds; they sell credit default swaps. These are sold not only in New York but also in The Netherlands. The spreads had grown wide until HSBC stepped in. That day in London, Sir John's speechwriter coined a phrase: a marriage of a premier deposit gatherer with one of the top asset gatherers in the U.S. of A.. This last, to the uninitiated, meant loans: debts are assets held by banks. Household reports securitization trust data that's distorted as a fun-house mirror by the repeated flipping of seniors in storefronts. Since value's determined by perception not reality, what does it matter?

There are well-schooled minds that are watching this deal. From Wharton and the LSE, those in the know say the merger makes sense. What was near junk bond status is now in the mainstream. They measure these things in bps or basis points. The Lord Marshall has spoken and the spreads are getting tight. Now if only these groups who demand their pound of flesh could be arrested, junk would become gold and they'd all get a bonus.

Some of these hotshots place calls to the storefront. They want, they say, to understand the advocates' concerns. Predatory lending is too vague: what's the status of the RAL litigation, they want to know. Someone should sue. Will it be a national story? Only if the national press declares it so. What power they have, the editors of the Journal and the New York Times. The former writes on RALS but does not mention Household. The latter once did but has stopped. The scribes, and their masters behind them, have declared the deal good. A macro-economist in Bermuda calls to schmooze. His accent is German; the rum punch is good. It's a bet on the future, he says. It's a profoundly hopeful thing.

Who then *are* these bitter ones who remain caught in the past? Doesn't the settlement wash away all Household's sins? Why not take a payment and get on the bandwagon? The elderly couple is not at the table. They're fodder for all these discussions. Their beat homes are the b in bps.

38.

The wide canyon of Park Avenue is a walk of trading shame. We once served papers here, copies of complaints on Chase's twitching-faced flak. He was rushed; his limousine was triple-parked outside. They were buying Advanta, another hard lender which began its game with teachers. Once its loans were mixed into a wider loan they smelled clean. The sidewalks of Park Avenue are hosed down at midnight. The water is heated and steams with absolution's humidity.

Of Chase's flak it must be said: the man is a racist. This term we try to not abuse. But when first challenged, he summoned us down to his then-office near Wall Street. There were sodas and ice, a stack of sandwiches; there were business cards like onion skin translucent. The well-greased door was closed and twitch-face drew a line. "We will not," he said, "engage in quota lending. We just don't do it."

But in fact a quota is just what they had. To make their record better, they offered no-money-loan loans for a month in Buffalo. When a number deemed sufficient was reached, the program was off. "We've been vindicated," Mr. Twitch declared. Since then it's been only war.

But not always uninvited: once we ate quail, with the nicer flak of Bankers Trust. Two men in a room; the waiter deemed of other species. "You kicked their ass good," he told me. The Partnership, he meant: the New York City Housing Partnership and its Margaret Thacher-like strongman the wild Kathy Wylde. She defended a bank that Inner City attacked. She got twenty-two groups to denounce the squatting group that thought it knew banking. And all for naught: the bank, Dime Savings, settled. It opened a branch in The Bronx. Squatters or not, the branch is still there. Kathy Wylde now sucks up to Henry K. Kravis, the LBO king. Bankers Trust was bought by Deutsche Bank, after coming near failing. There will be no more quail with this flak. Even the boardroom is gone, moved downtown before the planes arrived. Atta mistook the tallest for power. Park Avenue is the nerve center: the water is heated by the wires beneath. Trillions of dollars flow under the

street.   Perhaps the cables are under the Concourse.   In the Bronx bearded men steal copper from the Metro-North.   From time to time they die and it goes unreported.   They are digging for the wrong wires.   The pipes with the money are more
carefully buried.

39.

The cover-up for the Household's and Citi's of the world are the small ones: miniscule lenders who are easily sued.   The New York Banking Department, from whose Web site George Pataki smiles smugly, has scalps on its walls.   Delta Funding settled first; then Roslyn then the truly small.   One was called Anvil: its pitchman bought half-hour slots on the cable.   He chanted with extras in a church-like half-circle: you can own your own home!   Do not support your landlord!   Just fill out this form and deposit half a thousand dollars.   Then Anvil made no loans.   It had, in fact, no money to lend.   The application fees disappeared, and with them Anvil and its founder.   Ever pro-active, the Department then sued.   Cease and desist.   But Anvil had already fleeced and split.

On the other, leftern coast, the cipher was PinnFund.   A shyster with an MBA and a taste for used-up porn stars offered mortgage loans. The banks now called Mizuho, they financed the PinnFund.   The ones impaled, they were mostly of color.   Off-color jokes in the Financial Times; an SEC indictment and a flight to warmer climes.   How funny, this PinnFund, and Anvil before it.   And yet also what a sideshow.   If Citigroup does it, why can't Anvil too?   Well, Citi has Rubin; Citi has Clinton's flak John Podesta.   Anvil had only its heavy cross to bear.   It was like shooting a silver fish in a barrel; Pataki shot first but Spitzer shot better.   Then they both moved on.   They needed Citi's money to run their next campaigns.   The choice of targets is not rocket-science.   Those who move slow and can't pay the toll take the heat.   Next question.
* * *
The question is recusal.   The New York Superintendent of Banks has recused herself from decision-making on HSBC's applications to acquire Household.   The basis of the recusal is that the Superintendent's husband is a managing director at Goldman Sachs, which is Household's investment bank.   But the Superintendent did *not* recuse herself from negotiating or finalizing this Settlement, despite the fact that Household

formally retained Goldman Sachs, on May 1, 2002, to find it a buyer. This required a settlement, and the cheaper the better. ICP raises it, including to the New York State Ethics Commission. It is not popular. But it is a question.

40.

Even in time of war, soldiers' homes are foreclosed on. They start with the veterans but once that pool is dry they shift their action to active servicemen. Proclaiming its patriotism, Household gives two million dollars to the University of Maryland, to set up the Household Military Financial Education Resource Center. It will deliver courses and programs to U.S. troops and their dependents in 28 foreign countries; it is, Household says, "designed to meet the special needs of military personnel and their families." The only down-side is the service revolver. The Department of Defense, its domestic safeguards are porous. Perhaps they'll even endorse Household Finance -- some unions have.

The AFL-CIO is a partner of Household's. The Union Privilege card was something HSBC wanted. The private label too: thirty percent interest on furniture and garden tools. First you suck the leaf-blower up, then through that, the house. It's all written on mouse pads, like Moses' tablets. The key thing's to hide them when examiners come. In an affidavit filed by the Federal Trade Commission, an employee of CitiFinancial, Michelle Handzel, says just this. Still the bank regulators don't care. They'd rather not see the mouse pad, it seems. Inner City Press raises all of these issues to the Federal Reserve against Citigroup's application to buy Golden State Bancorp. It goes on for months, a new round of exhibits each Monday. The Fed asks ten sets of questions, but the answers are all blacked-out. They've got a secret thing going on, Citi and the Fed. The Fed hauls off and approves, saying only that their on-site examination of CitiFinancial will continue, expanded now to include credit insurance sales practices.

Three Fed lawyers travel south for depositions. Only ex-employees will talk: two were fired, and one left voluntarily. This last, he sold insurance to an eighty year old woman on a ladder. The woman wasn't on the ladder: the insurance was. Another employee exposes this and is fired for her troubles. It's called a suspension so she can't get unemployment. The second one treated this way sues and wins: she wins her unemployment. The Citi colossus moves on. They've got bigger problems, named Grubman and Enron. There's Dynagy and WorldCom, too. They take a billion dollar charge. The stock goes up. The test is almost over, Citi's Number Two Man Chuck Prince is heard to say. He and Sandy joke about buying drinks for all employees. But not the drones at CitiFinancial. For them there are suspensions; there are lock-outs and browbeatings. As with the borrowers, it depends which door of the Citi you enter. Start low, end low. It is brutal, and Swanker-Spitzer doesn't care. Too Big To Fail is sometimes translated as Too Big To Screw With. Foreplay and subpoena, yes. But when the settlement talks get serious, it's money that's screaming and not the victims.

41.

One might have thought that September 11, 2001, would have at least slowed the advance of predatory lending. But it did not. In the storefronts of Household and CitiFinancial, it was spun into an opportunity to sell more insurance. At Household's corporate campus in Prospect Heights, Illinois, William Aldinger ranted at the snot-nosed analysts who drove his stock price down. Soon he would take a sterner approach to these quants: "Who are *you*," he'd confront them, "to question how we serve our customers? They have bumps in the road, a car that dies, or a relative on the way out -- and we refi the loans. We charge them more because we take more risk, simple as that."

Aldinger could play the Horatio Alger song-and-dance. He'd been born in Brooklyn; later he'd tell reporters that On the Waterfront captured his childhood. He went to Baruch College; he got a job at U.S. Trust and then Citibank. Soon came a promotion to Wells Fargo, reporting directly to the CEO Carl Reichardt. What he dealt in was rich people's money: on the waterfront, yes,, but San Tropez and not Red Hook. In 1994, destiny called him: Household Finance needed a turn-around specialist. He decamped to the suburbs of Chicago, kicked out the deadwood like the football coach Bear Bryant. Then the time came to begin his acquisitions. Transamerica in '97, and also ACC. Then the big one: Beneficial Finance, which competed with Household in strip malls and storefronts.

Only one protest was filed: hotheads from The Bronx by the name of ICP. Bill dispatched a lawyer by the name of Ken Robins.

They met at a law firm in midtown Manhattan and soon struck a deal: Household committed to make normal-rate loans, $3 billion of them to the low-and-mod segment. The Office of Thrift Supervision soon gave approval. The so-called referral-up was called state of the art: offering people with good credit normal-priced loans. Whether it happened is not known. HSBC made a claim that HFC had no such product. They would carry that brand to the developing world, sure to make America and Britain new grateful friends with systemic loan sharking.

42.

If the CRA is law, why do these groups settle? ICP had decided that suing was better. It filed suit on U.S. Trust and Chase, then again on Chemical. Corporate lawyers filled the hallways of the Second Circuit Court of Appeals, begging to see Judge Miner. This group, they said in writing, was just trying to extort. Here is a letter from Thomas D. Barr:

"[B]oth banks would be at risk for millions of dollars and many thousands of individuals would suffer losses and inconvenience of a very major sort... There are serious questions concerning Mr. Lee and his colleagues' standing, of their status to represent whomever it is they may represent since, to the best of our knowledge, none of them is a lawyer... This merger has nothing to do with Mr. Lee or his colleagues or any complaints they may have, except that the threatened harm by the request of a stay provides a measure of leverage which Mr. Lee, *et al.*, may be seeking to obtain, albeit that leverage in some sense may aid plaintiffs in obtaining what they apparently believe to be legitimate social goals... I am authorized to state that Mr. Douglas B. Jordan, representing the Federal Reserve Board, has read this and joins with me in asking the Court to deny the application for a stay in all respects. We will, of course, do our best to get a copy of this letter into Mr. Lee's hands and will be available in the court house this afternoon at 2:00 should your Honor wish to hear from us. Respectfully yours, Thomas D. Barr."

It's from Cravath, Swaine & Moore; Judge Miner pays attention. The stay is denied and the case scheduled for briefing. When the day for argument comes, behind the high wooden bench sits Ellsworth A. Van Graafeiland. There are questions of standing; there are questions of harm. Later there is a decision, which puts the CRA in its place: it is "amorphous" and obtuse, a "merely precatory" statute. The CRA, he writes, is not "a directive to undertake any particular program or to provide credit to any particular individual... It is impossible to discern ... the effects' of any past injury or to support a finding of impending future injury... It is important that the issues arising out of the several mergers finally be disposed of."

Not only Chase's mergers, but ICP and the CRA are disposed of: twenty-six pages, straight to the law books. Thereafter, community groups settled for what they can. Household will refer-up? Oh that it were so. Now there will be only war, comments that attack the regulators as much as the banks, Fair Finance Watching.

43.

One can try other judges, and ICP did. The Tenth Circuit in Denver, against NationsBank and Boatmen's Bancshares. The biggest firm in Denver is hired to oppose. Judge Lucero sides with them; appeal to the Supremes comes next. Justice Kennedy will not suggest a grant of cert. Later the D.C. Circuit rules the same way: three strikes and you're out. A law without a remedy is not a law, some say. American law is about the individual, about concrete harm that can be paid-for and absolved. So it is with Household, which help H&R Block settle the class actions they choose. Judge Richard Posner, reading late in the night not far from Prospect Heights, sees through the smoke screen [*see* 288 F.3d 277 (2002), and Chapterette 10, *above*].

Aldinger grumbles; a nicer judge in rural Texas is found. For HSBC to buy, it all must look clean. Household starts a new bonus program: $400 to each account executive who re-writes a delinquent loan. It is raised to the regulators; it is raised to the SEC. Nobody cares, at least initially. A British reporter is asked: what's the beef? If the re-write helps the customer, why do you care? Because once the deal is done, things will only get worse.

Then, out of the blue, it seems, the SEC announces a cease-and-desist order against Household, accusing it of false and misleading reporting of loan status. The SEC -- Release Number 47528 under the Securities Act of 1934 -- says that its investigation is "ongoing." But Household claims it's only ongoing as to "others," whom it does not define. Could it be Aldo? No one will say until Aldo gets paid. One can imagine already the subsequent release: to pursue other opportunities, to spend time with family. What kind of family spends time with a loan shark? A family that likes an indoor swimming pool. A school of loan sharks, endowed by HFC.

44.

Already hidden behind H&R Block, Household creates yet another veil. A California bank, Imperial Capital, will now on paper make the loans. Household will buy them, using the high rate as entrée for more debilitating loans. The Federal Reserve turns a blind eye as always. They placate bond traders with rate cuts, but as to the others it's caveat emptor.

On the edge of Babe Ruth Plaza sits an H&R Block. The sign says Rapid Refund,™ but it's a loan from Beneficial. Four doors down is a branch that CRA opened: it was then called Dime Savings and is now Washington Mutual. WaMu, too, has its talons in subprime. Its branch name is Long Beach. Its rates reach forty percent. A day before snow, the BBC comes. They will document the work of ICP: the branch that HSBC closed, this one that Dime Savings opened. Later in London, a guest's in the studio: it's Susan Rice from old NatWest, nor flaking in Scotland for Lloyds TSB. "My old bank," she says, "opened a branch in The Bronx without any pressure." It is a lie, but the Atlantic is wide.

The Bronx has been lied to for decades, it seems. Robert Moses built a highway, and sixty thousand families were homeless. Under Reagan some contracts were given to Wedtech: the ladder of opportunity turned out to be a fraud. The last generation of Riverdale boys -- Stanley Friedman, Stanley Simon, and from Throgs Neck, Biaggi -- they all went to jail. The new boss was Freddie, who sold The Bronx to slumlords. Later Amadou Diallo got shot. Forty one times, no mistake but no guilt either. The D.A. lost the case but didn't lose his job. So it goes in The Bronx. More than elsewhere, in The Bronx it is true that the law is a whore.

45.

There's a man from Citigroup whose name is Martin Wong. He works for the Prince of darkness, but always with a smile. In Jefferson City, Missouri, he dodged cross-examination. Not as boldly as the

Prince down in Dover, but not without effect, not without evasion. When you're work for Sandy, you do what you're told. High over Queens he ate canapés and laughed. "I'm in something cleaner now," he said. "I specialize in privacy." His real job is pay-offs. In Alabama, it's said, he encouraged class actions. Lawyers who'd settle for cents on the dollar, in exchange for a nice padded fee. In the play-out of the *Morales* case, it's all on display. In briefs filed before the ironically-named fairness hearing, the lawyers submit their bills. But first they argue:

> "The Inner City Press / Community on the Move objects to the proposed settlement primarily because it does not include injunctive relief to ensure that the same 'packing' and 'flipping' practices at issue in the litigation do no continue or reoccur. Specifically, the objector contends, there is no assurance that the predatory lending practices at issue in the litigation will [not] continue, under the CitiFinancial name, unless the settlement includes an order for injunctive relief... Plaintiffs respond that the primary injunctive relief sought by the litigation, an order enjoining defendants from engaging in deceptive solicitation and/or sale of loans or add-on products, was satisfied in advance of the parties' settlement. Specifically, since the acquisition of The Associates in November 2000, Citigroup, Inc., has voluntarily adopted a series of consumer-oriented initiatives that address concerns raised by Plaintiffs, the FTC and others regarding The Associates' credit insurance and refinancing practices. As the $240 million settlement was obtained in conjunction with a voluntary adoption of a 'best practices' policy by Associates' successor, Plaintiffs respond that the proposed settlement is fair, adequate, and reasonably considers the injunctive relief obtained."

Here a slew of class action firms say that Citigroup's non-binding and weak "voluntary" reforms are enough for them. Apparently, *they* will enforce Citigroup's compliance with its vague promises -- once they've been paid, of course. It's take-the-money-and-run time. In a separate brief, the plaintiffs' lawyers defend their proposed $23 million fee. They state that Citigroup "acknowledged the substantial contribution that Plaintiffs made in connection with their settlement with the FTC by stating to the mediators that at least $100 million of the $215 million settlement with the FTC was attributable to Plaintiffs' Counsel." The real deal? Citigroup was willing to pay more to the FTC so that it could get the abusively broad release of claims by victim that the $120-a-head *Morales* settlement provides.

The *Morales* lawyers set their fees at up to $690 an hour -- and $155 an hour for a "Summer Law Clerk." Another firm charges $875 for two-and-a-half hours of "[e]xtensive internet investigation of allegations that Citigroup has been involved in predatory lending practices." Inner City Press' web site at least is lucrative to someone. The firm charges $350 an hour for travel time. They're getting paid $350 an hour for surfing the Internet -- why *not* for sleeping on a train down the coast?

* * *

At Citigroup, law and lobbying go hand-in-hand. Chuck Prince praises Oxley; the feeling is mutual. Martin Wong knows Gifford Miller. At City Hall he tweaks the city's ordinance. Soon a Bushite is hired, then the head-man from the IMF. It's not what you know but who you know. Household doesn't know this: they get a second-rate regulator from the Keystone State, James Kauffman; they get a played-out Congressman from upstate New York. These press releases do not grab attention. Like HSBC they are the soul of discretion.

In Britain, you see, the peers -- members of the House of Lords -- freely sit on corporate boards. HSBC has three of them, a record. There's the Baroness Dunn, who from 1997 into 2002 was on the board of an ex-arms manufacturer turned telecom disaster, Marconi plc. HSBC's other deputy chairman, Sir Brian Moffat, is the chairman of the steel company Corus, formed from the cold-fusion of the Hoogovens group of the Netherlands and British Steel -- then they brought in "Sir Brian... the dour chairman who once said he was more interested in making money than steel." Steely Sir Brian, hungry for Household. It's positively medieval.

46.

What makes these Lords and Sirs believe that they can harness Household? They bought banks on the cheap in Brazil; they negotiated-down the price of Republic after its dirty business in the former USSR. Subprime, then, is a piece of cake, they think. They can bring in deposits from all over the world to fund these high-cost loans. The watchers of finance devise a new idea: to hit each and every HSBC acquisition proposal, wherever it may be. For example in Singapore: just after the Household announcement, HSBC cuts a deal to buy Keppel insurance. There are laws on the site of the Monetary Authority of Singapore, something about the need for High Court approval. A comment's prepared and faxed off in the night. The Sirs will be far less than happy. They will call it extortion; they will spin their Rolodex to G, for Gramm. Texas senator Gramm, long the friend and beneficiary of right-wing banks. Gramm almost killed the CRA. But now he is gone, out through the revolving door, to vice chair the Swiss bank UBS. He can no longer help. Now he and UBS, like HSBC, are just targets. It is more lucrative but not without its frustrations. There's no subpoena power. One has to shuck and jive, trying to make up for the dive in Enron's stock. The cash-in from The Hill is an old story: ask Bob Dole. Ask Connie Mack, who flacks for Household. The bully pulpit's not portable.

* * *

Still Household tries, or claims it does. When the Washington Department of Financial Institutions looked into complaints of rate and terms misquoted, not only did Household try to get the exam report sealed -- it also conducted its own investigation. Its spin was that the EZ-Pay worksheets has never been authorized. Employees faxed them to each other because they made the sales so easy. From Prospect Heights Bill Aldinger ordered each and every copy destroyed. Then on a conference call with analysts he claimed that these problems were all in the past.

At least Aldinger answered the question, however incompletely. Citigroup, due to its size, does not hold calls on these matters. When Inner City Press raised some problems from South Carolina, Citi stonewalled, even reporters. A woman from Reuters, a guy from the Financial Times -- to each of them, Citi's main flak Leah Johnson said "ICP's crazy," and left it at that. She confirmed, however, that they'd sent a Skadden Arps attorney down. His name was Mitch Ettinger; in his first call to the ex-employees he noted that he'd defended Clinton against Paula Jones. "You could look it up," he said. Later in Charleston he threatened to sue them. "You've signed an agreement to never disparage," he reminded them. "You'll pay attorneys fees too" -- his. Some money changed hands, to the ex-employees, and the problem went away. The only trace was a squib in the American Banker of July 30, 2001, *Citi Corroborates Two Allegations*:

Citigroup Inc. has acknowledged that at least some of a former employee's claims of unfair lending practices at its subprime unit, CitiFinancial Mortgage, have been confirmed. The allegations, in an affidavit signed by former loan officer Steven Toomey, are that at least one Charleston, S.C., CitiFinancial office had a policy of not giving borrowers legally required disclosures in a timely manner, that employees there regularly forged borrowers' signatures on legal documents, and that loan officers were instructed to avoid telling potential borrowers about points and fees on loans.

In response to repeated phone and e-mail requests for comment, Citigroup spokeswoman Leah Johnson issued a statement Thursday that reads in part: "We interviewed Mr. Toomey, and among the many allegations he described, we were able to corroborate only two isolated incidents and have taken appropriate corrective action." She would not answer questions about what specific activities had been corroborated or what corrective action had been taken. However, Ms. Johnson confirmed that Citigroup had accepted the resignation of a manager mentioned in the Toomey affidavit, Tim Delapaz, on July 25.

Citigroup, in a statement July 9, tried to play down Mr. Toomey's allegations, saying that he had worked for CitiFinancial a short time and "only in the last few weeks raised issues related to branch sales practices when he concluded that the company would not pay him monies that he demanded to resolve an employment dispute."

Mr. Toomey's affidavit was taken by Matthew Lee, the executive director of Inner City Press/Community on the Move, a fair-housing activist organization in New York City. Mr. Lee, who said he has interviewed numerous former CitiFinancial employees, has alleged that several were told they had to sign nondisparagement agreements with the company as a condition for receiving their final paychecks.

A copy of one such agreement, obtained by American Banker, bars the former employee from making "any statements to any person regarding the company and its agents of a derogatory nature or which disparages the reputation, business, or integrity of the company or any of the executives or employees of the company." It also contains a clause barring the former employee from disclosing the agreement. Ms. Johnson would not comment on the circumstances under which employees were asked to sign the nondisparagement agreements.

47.

The big guys buy silence; only the little guys' cases actually make it to trial. Take, for example, Capitol City Mortgage in Washington, D.C.. They got sued; while it was pending, they moved the assets out. Bush II's Justice Department wrung its hands and said, "We tried." Rather like the attorneys general of the many states on Household. We did our best, said Connecticut's Blumenthal. Spitzer never had to answer. The Iowa staffer fumes still. "But we're on the same side," Inner City is told. "Why attack them?" Because they had leverage and wasted it. It was a predatory lending settlement that flew by night. They knew it and they didn't care. So Inner City took its venom to Asia.

While HSBC shucked and jived in its attempt to buy Household, its hungers elsewhere were slaked. On December 20 from Hong Kong it announced a deal for Keppel Insurance of Singapore. Though the wonders of Google, Inner City saw the news; while snow fell it stewed and fermented. The day after Christmas, Inner City lashed out: a twenty page fax to the Monetary Authority of Singapore, asking them to review the prospective financial strength of HSBC. Predatory lending, as an issue, was going global. In England they spoke of the Provident door-knockers; in Hong Kong it's JCG Finance. Maids from the Philippines refinance their debts to their snakeheads. As collateral, their passports are taken. It's an ugly business that Citi and HSBC Household want to rationalize, in both meanings of that word. There's a coming new age of reason; there's coming a season on laminated loan sharks. And so onto Kenya:

Subj: Predatory lending in Kenya via takeover by HSBC of Equator Bank
Date: 2/28/03 1:40:48 AM Eastern Standard Time
To: [ICP / Fair Finance Watch]

We appreciate the trouble you took to put the long dossier together and will take full cognizance of your warning about the practice of predatory lending. Thank you very much for your warning.

Patrick N. Ndwiga, Manager, Bank Supervision, CENTRAL BANK OF KENYA

Never let it be said the alarm wasn't raised.

48.

What's needed, of course, is the background on cases. Anyone can complain -- but where are the facts? Perhaps at the interstices of sealed depositions. Here's Household, from Luna versus HFC in the Western District of Washington, 02-CV-1635:

Q: Were you ever told to destroy such unauthorized worksheets or comparison charts?

A: It depends on what you mean by the unauthorized comparison charts.

Q: Have you ever destroyed or shredded worksheets or comparison charts any that that you've been a Household employee?

A: Yes....

Q: Do you believe that the decision to go paperless was an attempt to cover up those documents where customers had been told about the effective interest rate, comparable interest rate or equivalent interest rate?

MR. PAYSON: Objection, calls for speculation.

A: I don't know either way.

* * *

In the spring of 2002, Inner City hit an application by Option One and its parent H&R Block. The former does mortgages at twenty percent; the latter does tax loan at rates of four hundred, in partnership with none other than Household's Beneficial Finance. This is called advocate's synergy: the use of documents from one proceeding in another. By the savvy use of FOIA, Inner City obtained a list of litigation against Block and Benny. This confidential exhibit referred to refers to "New York City Department of Consumer Affairs Litigation" (Notice of Violation Case #CL 59286, April 2001); JTH, Inc., d/b/a Liberty Tax Services, et al. v. H&R Block Eastern Tax Services, Inc., *et al.*, a "suit pending in the federal courts in Virginia since February 2000;" and states that "[f]our separate lawsuits have been filed against the Company since the release of the Fourth Circuit decision in the JTH case noted above. They are pending in the United States District Court for the Eastern District of Virginia."

Despite this Virginia nexus, soon after came a letter on pretty sky-blue stationary from the Richmond office of Virginia's senior assistant attorney general for consumer litigation. A bone is thrown to ICP: "You raise important questions, which I believe are best addressed in the context of the state and federal regulatory proceedings related to approval of that transaction." But there was no Virginia proceeding, and at the federal level there was only the Comptroller of the Currency, a Clintonite hold-over trying to keep his position by providing relief to the loan sharks. All praise to the double-faced play-out of the dual banking system.

49.

To meet with Option One was required. They'd complained that Inner City was dodging, and so a sit-down was set. In a windowless room of a law firm in midtown, after a pungent lunch on a metal chair in Bryant Park. Option One came with PowerPoint;™ they came with a video that announced their best practices. As to how and why they lent, there were very few answers. Later there were Christmas cards, from Option One and its lawyer. Ameriquest also sent one, with an "Esq." in the midst of the snowy winter scene it depicted. From Household only silence. There was some fight-back in the works.

* * *

But first, of course, the pay-offs. When HSBC filed its preliminary proxy statement with the SEC on December 20, the media quickly seized on Aldinger's bonus. He'd get ten million dollars if the merger was approved. Then five point five for each of the next two years, on top of his six million salary, and some undefined severance package he's also be collecting on. Seven other Householders also got paid. But it was Aldo, as they called him, who came under fire.

"Aldo sold us out!" e-screamed the Household ex-employees on their list serv.

"They think he's a genius," said another, more quietly. "They think he was tried in the press and still was never found guilty."

Conspiracy theories abounded, of how Aldo has feathered his nest. "You can't do anything to stop it," one resigned blogger said. "So why not just enjoy your holiday?"

Aldo, the moniker, had many connotations. There was Italian P.M. Aldo Moro, kidnapped and shot by the Red Brigades. Perhaps more pertinent, there's the old cartoon of a big-nosed man in a quickly-sketched crowd: "Where's (W)Aldo?" And where *was* Aldo, anyway? Could it be that he didn't exist, that he'd died yet lived in on quotes in Household's press releases? In October Oh-Two, he'd apologized to customers. He'd been heard on a conference call, that day and a month later announcing the deal. But perhaps it had been pre-recorded; perhaps that's why they never filed the transcript with the SEC. But who, one wondered, would cash those huge checks?

50.

Back in the storefronts, the options are narrower. The sale of credit insurance, on which the companies rarely have to pay, is lucrative. Employees' bonus, at Household and Citi, ride on the sale of the product. Both tell the regulators that insurance is entirely voluntary. But at the point of sale, this is not true. Citi, for example, instructs in a memo: Ask the customer how much they can pay, then design a protected product to fit that need. The loan is presented with insurance included. They've already said they could pay this much a month: so where's the beef? If push comes to shove, there's always the old stand-by: you can't get the loan without insurance. Or, the loan can only close today if you take it as written. It works like a charm, whatever the small-font type disclosures say to the contrary.

The most absurd sale is insurance on ladders. Leaf-blower, lawnmowers, even fishing rods and reels. In April Oh Two in vast Carnagie Hall, Inner City asked Sandy about these fishing rods. Sandy

turned red, redder than his tie. He did not respond; he referred to
Chuckles Prince. Only later, on July 18, did the Wall Street Journal get
Citi's response:

When it makes a personal loan, CitiFinancial often asks the holders
of personal loans to provide collateral. In some cases, according to
CitiFinancial documents filed by Inner City Press, that collateral
includes fishing lures and tackle boxes, record albums, tents,
sleeping bags and lanterns -- items that CitiFinancial would almost
certainly never bother to collect in the event of a borrower's default.
Yet insurance is sold on the collateral in case it is damaged or lost.
"It's predatory: This insurance product has no rationale, because it's
not credible that someone would want to have their loan paid with
their leaf-blower," said Matthew Lee, executive director of the Fair
Finance Watch project at Inner City Press. "Citigroup has not lived
up to the subprime lending reforms it announced after acquiring
Associates."

Citigroup officials concede seizing such collateral would be more
hassle than it's worth. But they say providing such collateral on loans
has a purpose -- "to make the borrower more responsible for paying
the loan back," says Ajay Banga, Citigroup's business head of
consumer lending.

51.

Those who make money on the stock only care if the scam will
continue. Of Aldo they asked, how much will the settlement cost you
per share? Aldo's answer seemed anachronistic. "Barely a dime," he
said. "Whatever we give up in points and fees we can make up in rate."
"What about mandatory arbitration? I mean, if all these people
can sue you, it's sure to cost--"
"It never came up," Also cut it. He'd had the AGs in this pocket,
as he now had the analysts. And little did they know that the end-game
was in place. Sir John and his factotum Nasr were sniffing around; the
very day of the settlement they began final due diligence. "It'll all work
out," Aldo said. "You'll see."
What was in the AGs' staffers' minds, we still do not know.
While Household had to purport to disclose the background to the

merger, the government prosecutors are shrouded in secrecy. "You're assuming a lot," Ms. Iowa said. "I'm drowning in other cases," said Mr. Washington. A staffer from New York cut straight to the chase: "We are *not* going to reopen the settlement. We just are not." But why not? Their word was their bond, apparently. It seems laughable, in these Enron times. Unnecessary, too: the announcement of the merger was a "material" change, under any definition. As one arb put it, though, the ABs had already gotten good press. What more could be gained? They might even be accused of jeopardizing the economic recovery. No, there was no angle in defending consumers, in taking a second bite at the apple. Get in, get out; declare victory. Who'll even know that you could have gotten more? Anyone that reads the proxy. But who reads these things, that clot up the servers of the SEC's Edgar? On airplanes, the fodder is thrillers: legal and now even financial. As in horror films, camera and audience identify with the doer, and not the victim.

52.

Charlotte, city perennially on the cusp, played a big role in subprime. Here it was that NationsBank's Hugh McColl pulled the trigger on Chrysler First, then called it NationsCredit. Later he'd buy Equicredit and later still, retire. Here also, First Union's Ed Crutchfield made his ill-fated deal for the Money Store. It's a city of pawnshops and check cashing shops. It's a very centered city: from nearly every point one can see the Bank of America tower, the so-called Taj McColl. Glittering jagged and angry over a foreground of boarded-up factories; rising high and lying over forgotten expanses of shotgun shacks; spry and cosmopolitan at the end of a string of Waffle Houses on South Boulevard.

Charlotte was founded in 1769. Two Indian trading paths crossed here, Tryon and Trade. During the Revolutionary War, General Cornwallis called Charlotteans hornets, and they've clung to this image since, most recently as the mascot of their doomed-and-departed pro basketball team. In 1983, Charlotte became a regional hub for airplane flights. They built a football stadium in the 1990s, Home of the Carolina Panthers. It comes to life precisely eight times a year. Nine, if the Panthers make the playoffs. It's, past sad factories with their windows smashed, quiet neighborhoods with a few homes boarded-up. In a strip mall there are payday loans; there's an outlet for Trojan Labor, "workers when you need them." And when you don't need them, no workers. It's very convenient, unless you're a worker.

South Boulevard is a string of strip malls selling Italian tiles for the bathroom, a Waffle House with its tall yellow sign, a Cash America pawnshop. Downtown there's a bus station; there's a historical sign-post about Stonewall Jackson, and an in-land Confederate Navy Yard that made ordnance for the Confederate troops. Now there's a Starbucks; a performance center named for the heir of Liquid Wrench and Gunk, a crafts museum and a public library where the Internet runs free. Year-old banking books are for sale for a quarter. Bland jazz seeps from the bar of the Dunhill Hotel. Four blocks west on Trade, there are cheaper accommodations. A five-story Travelodge with its hallways outside, across from the Greyhound bus station and the Presto Grill. Presto! Down the hill, cowering under the banks' towers, is the two-story

Charlotte branch of the Federal Reserve Bank of Richmond. The bank examiners desperately want to get a job up the hill, and they'll sweep problems under the rug to accomplish their goals. Derivatives fiascoes in Singapore? No problem. Predatory lending in Greensboro? No problem. Hire me and let me swill Starbucks in the clouds, high over Piedmont, and all problems will disappear.

53.

Beyond the total deregulation of banking, privacy too was a component of the repeal of the Glass-Steagall Act. Opt-in, opt-out: it was an arcane issue, followed most closely by washed-up advocates and a combed-over Senator from Alabama. This was all pre-Nine Eleven; now with face-recognition technology and the Carnivore, Chinese walls for telemarketers seem less important.

The purpose of Gramm, Leach & Bliley -- like Crosby, Stills & Nash, only older -- was to let Citi-Travelers stand and encourage more mergers. Schwab bought U.S. Trust; various banks got into private equity. Citigroup bought auto parts; Bank One bought a submarine factory and even Polaroid. Then a recession, the fall of the Towers - the law was hardly used. Phil Gramm cashed out to the Swiss Bank UBS; Jim Leach was term-limited and retired elsewhere in his sweater. Even Bliley left. It was the man from Alabama who took the reins, and where he'd drive, nobody knew.

In Birmingham they sue and chew tobacco. They sue State Farm for using used auto parts in repairs. They sue the financier of satellite TV dishes; they sue anything that moves. There are calls for tort reform. Even Sixty Minutes tries to pile-on the jurors (so much for populism). But it's hardly anti-business down Birmingham way. When Inner City took a shot at AmSouth, it was reported on A.P.. Within a day, the AmSoutherners had summoned local editors and begun their counter-spin. Later they'd quietly settle race discrimination charges. None of it mattered. They expanded into Florida. The South shall rise again.

* * *

What was once the Third World is now the Global South. In part it's p.c. -- Third World is a stigma -- and in part it's the implosion of the second, Soviet, world. The South is not geography. Australia, for example, is below Indonesia but much higher in income. Like emerging markets, it's a buzzword. It's where Citigroup is, and where HSBC wants to take Household. Though they deny it: following the filing in Chapterette 46, the Straits Times quotes HSBC spokesman Goh Kong Aik that "the proposed acquisition of Household International has no bearing on our business in Singapore. The concerns expressed by ICP relate entirely to Household's operations within the US, where they are being considered by regulators responsible for reviewing the acquisition. Household has no operations in Singapore." But that's only for now.

54.

Delaware is next. The conflicted counsel for the Department Insurance -- which he insists on calling the "DID" -- opposes the inclusion in the DID's record of documents ICP's submitted concerning real-time complaints against Household, buck-passing of predatory credit insurance issues from the DID to the Delaware Banking Department, and inconsistencies in the sworn affidavits of Sir John Bond, Youssef Nasr and HSBC executive Timothy O'Brien. But there's more: DID's brief argues that Insurance Commissioner Donna Lee Williams' acceptance of campaign contributions from Household should *not* require her recusal from decision-making. But there's a old statute, 18 Del. C. §2304(6)a, which says that "no insurer... shall directly or indirectly pay or use, or offer, consent or agree to pay or use, any money or property for or in aid of any candidate for the office of Insurance Commissioner of the State." Household has done just this; the contribution was outright illegal. These things, however, can be made to go away.

* * *

HSBC's chairman Sir John Bond's said that HSBC will export Household's model to the 81 countries where HSBC does business, including Singapore. Household's wanted to expand globally but hasn't had the funding to do so, said Sir John. Enter the dragon. Before year-end of '02, the process begins: on Dec. 30, Household International Europe proposed to acquire a bank license in Poland, a type of expansion of which Household has sworn-off in the months and years prior to its HSBC announcement.

The Strait Times continues, "the Monetary Authority of Singapore (MAS), which received ICP's concerns over the Keppel acquisition, declined to comment on the matter. In a reply to queries, a spokesman said: 'MAS does not, as a matter of policy, comment on correspondence concerning financial institutions.' However, an official source said that at least one ICP concern - that deposits (insurance premiums) taken from one country may be used to fund loans in another - is prohibited under regulations." Sir John Bond has also repeatedly claimed that HSBC will deploy the deposits and profits it generates to fund Household's loans and Household's expansion. They have a sound byte: this is a marriage of a premier deposit collector -- the world's local bank -- with a premier "asset" generator. Asset is a fancy word for loan. The analysts opine that HSBC is now only lent-up to the tune of seventy percent 70% -- that is, 70% of deposits are in fact lent out; this figure would rise to ninety percent, they say. This balance is not accounted for by HSBC's un-lent deposits in the United States. So where *would* they come from?

* * *

In Poland, the game is quite sneaky. The Poland Business Review of December 9, 2002 reported that "Kredyt Bank president Stanislaw Pacuk told reporters Friday... to recoup losses, Kredyt Bank is **planning to sell the banking license** of its subsidiary, Polski Kredyt Bank, **to a British bank**." (Emphasis added.) Then on December 30, Reuters reported that "Household International, set to be acquired by Europe's largest bank HSBC, said on Monday that it planned to set up a retail network in Poland after buying a small local bank."

So HSBC is *already* using Household as a front, even before having the regulatory and shareholder approval to acquire Household. The Fair Finance Watchers ask the Polish Commission for Banking to inquire into the matter. The phone rates to Warsaw in the middle of the night are surprisingly cheap. And so Inner City Press calls Kredyt Bank and interviews its spokesman. He claims that HSBC has already taken-over Household; when asked whom to call at Household to confirm this, he says he has no contact there, only at HSBC. This is conveyed to The Times of London, which writes it along with a report on ICP's petitioning of HSBC's board of directors. The strategies are arrived at the night before they are implemented. A rule of guerrilla consumer advocacy is that one cannot only do what is already expected.

55.

And so at the eleventh hour, ICP writes to the Fed. There'll be an open meeting of its Consumer Advisory Council, where predatory lending is already of record. We go as camera-eye:

Fade in: holding pen in the lobby of the Federal Reserve's Martin Building, 20th and C Street. Upstairs the Fed's Consumer Advisory Council is meeting. By the metal detectors, name-tags await the pre-registered guests. These include the lobbyist for the subprime lender Option One, and Stacie McGinn of the Skadden Arps law firm, which represented Citigroup against charges of predatory lending. A quarter of an hour into the meeting, a Fed staffer named Ms. Featherstone escorts the observers to the Terrace Level meeting room. The CAC members are in a wide circle, with three of the Fed Governors: Gramlich, Bies and Bernanke.

Three days previous, Inner City Press has submitted a letter for distribution and action at this meeting. The letter asks the CAC to direct the Governors to make HSBC explain *why* it's appropriate to acquire Household and put Household's CEO Aldo in charge of HSBC's bank. The letter has been photocopied; there's a stack of copies on the table by the entranceway. But it doesn't come up during the hour-long discussion of predatory lending. There are questions from the surprisingly-large Governor Bies about state enforcement actions on brokers. The Fed's own duties are not discussed: a taboo. The Household issue, it seemed, was addressed in a non-open meeting on March 12. Fed staffer Dolores Smith has assured CAC members that the Fed will, on HSBC - Household, do what it did on Citigroup - Associates. And what was that? Allow the deal to be consummated, and *then* ask questions. That it makes little sense, in a post-Enron-Nine-Eleven world, is not brought up. There is a breakfast spread along the side wall, that even the visitors access. With the Federal Reserve, resources are not ever at issue.

Jump-cut to Scene #2, a composite: in meetings with various community groups, the chief counsel of the Office of the Comptroller of the Currency says that there's little that the OCC can or will do, since the HSBC application before it is technically about a credit card bank. But this was also true in Citigroup - Associates, and in *that* case, the OCC at least attended a public hearing on the deal, and Citigroup announced at least a few reforms. Neither has happened here -- the difference being, it seems, the intervening elections.

There's one further explanation: the Citi-Associates hearing was held by the New York Banking Department, but now that agency's in HSBC bag.   The Superintendent of Banks bungled forward with the narrow Household settlement, even as her husband's firm stood to make money.   Now she won't answer.   Her minions withhold documents, so ICP tries other states.   Indiana Deputy AG Coffey says it's interesting, but then himself withholding.   ICP appeals, to the state's Public Access Advisor.   In Utah, too, the envelope is stretched.   In old Salt Lake there's a hearing, on ICP's appeal.   Householders fly in from Chicago; an affidavit by James B. Kauffman says it's all a trade secret.   It'll all go online, and in the state's archive.   This is a law without dirty hands: the right of the people to every public record.   Even if usually once it's too late.

* * *

As it happens, there are Freedom of Information groupies, the "FOIA plaintiffs' bar," they call themselves.   It's National FOIA Day; the roof-top conference room of the Freedom Forum in Arlington, Virginia is packed.   The talk is of restrictions in access rationalized by terrorism.   But from the back of the room, Inner City Press has a question.   What about the states that say their FOIA laws are only for state residents?   From the podium there's outrage.   One eminence gris with balding pate has a theory: it violates the privileges and immunities clause of the U.S. Constitution!   He's asked to sue on this theory -- and indirectly, to stop the Household merger -- but can't, in the necessary time-frame.   Who can?

Most public interest lawyers of today see the government as their adversary.   Interventionist wars only increase this sense.   Who's fighting the corporations?   Who's using Regulation Fair Disclosure to undermine secrets?   The watchers of fair finance learn tricks, but only at the point of a gun.   Arbitrageurs demand that their phone calls be returned.   They suggest more cooperation with the acquirer: "you're losing your credibility with Wall Street."   Who knew that one had this?   And who cares?   They go along to get along.   "Focus on proposing reforms," they say.   That, too, can be done.

56.

Let's start with the basics: don't sell credit insurance on items that have already been insured.   It happens at both Household and Citi, and here's how: the customer needs -- needs! -- four thousand dollars. "We'll need security for the loan," she is told. A list is made: big screen TV, lawn mower, leaf blower. "But I already have homeowners' insurance." That's not good enough. She's free, of course, to get the insurance from another location. But that will take ten days. Sign here. There. It's done.

The reason the property list is requested is to sell the insurance. The company -- here Household and Citi -- has no intention of ever repossessing this junk. What would they do with it? Hold a yard sale, of collections of video tapes and thrice-dented mowers. The employees are paid based on how much they sell: insurance, incidental products, how high's the interest rate. And so another basic point: don't tie compensation to how much they sell, or how much they charge. As long as you do, the scams will continue. It's not rocket-science, but it's anti-American, we're told. The government won't intervene into these compensation schemes. Other countries, yes. But not this.

And so the rules as proposed look too late in the process. It's fun to lobby, some say. But if *this* is what democracy looks like -- boring seminars in the windowless basements of Washington hotels -- this is not the Holy Grail. Back to the barricades! Let there be class action lawsuits, let there be investigations! Let the sleazeballs who export this neo-loan sharking be pursued to the ends of the earth!

* * *

And that pursuit, for now, is the only option left. In the three days between HSBC's shareholders' meeting, the approvals fall sequentially like a hand in a rigged game of poker. Delaware Insurance devotes over forty-five pages, but nonetheless approves, following a flurry of rhetorical questions:

"Would it be a good idea to have a prophylactic examination of [Household's] two Delaware insurers in the near future? Given the Settlement and the Delaware Consent Judgment, should the examination be broadened to include the Department's Consumer Services and, for purposes of expert advice in establishing standards, possibly even the Fraud Bureau? Should the Department be concerned that its individual licensees are educated as to the Settlement and the Delaware Consent Judgment? ... Is Household Life a possible microcosm to examine the organization [Household International]?... Should Household have to account in better fashion as to its self-styled Best Practices on the insurance side of its business?"

Ohio Insurance is short and sweet but with the same result. New York Banking confines itself to three lines -- "we have approved." The next day, Superintendent McCaul resigns, "for various personal reasons." The arbs are in an uproar. It's all coming together, they say, adjusting their trading positions. From the storefront in The Bronx, a suit in filed in Ohio. But the court has no time to hear it, with the closing scheduled for the next afternoon. One stares at the Web cast from London.

Sir John Bond holds forth in a Canary Wharf conference room. He repeats his previous, inaccurate claim that 63% of Household's business is "prime." He procures his vote -- numerous HSBC directors hadn't even bothered to show up -- and at 5:02 p.m., the merger with Household is consummated, a paper filed with the Delaware Secretary of State. It's done.

57.

More documents trickle in, even "post-consummation," just as they'd planned it. There's a March 31, 2003, Open Records ruling from the Texas Attorney General's Office. ICP had asked that Office for documents about its settlement with Household, and about complaints against Household. Some responsive records were provided, but most were withheld at Household's request. ICP pursued the matter with Texas AG's Open Records Office, and on March 6, Household's outside counsel at Boudreaux, Leonard & Hammond in Houston submitted an eight-page letter claiming that virtually all documents were confidential. Household even withheld portions of its letter -- that is, of its argument -- from ICP. Household asserted three separate "exceptions" from the Open Records Act: "litigation or settlement negotiations involving the state," "confidential information," and, most broadly, trade secrets. For the documents it has numbered HHLD 0033-0079, Household stated that these "should be exempt from disclosure in their entirety because they contain confidential communications of settlement negotiations between Household and various state attorneys general and regulators, including those from the States of Washington, Wisconsin, Illinois, New York, Arizona and California. [REDACTED].. The litigation is pending...

Moreover, the information was provided with the understanding that it would remain confidential." The Texas Attorney General's Office, ruling three days after the merger was consummated, holds that "none of the submitted information may be withheld.. It is well-settled that the Public Information Act prevents a governmental body from promising to keep information confidential unless it is statutorily authorized to do so... Household states only that the submitted information should be protected from disclosure because it is critical to maintaining the company's competitive position in the market... Household has failed to demonstrate any of the factors necessary to establish a trade secrets claim. Since Household has failed to demonstrate that any of its claimed exceptions to disclosure apply, we conclude that the information at issue must be released." It's online, for no one, at www.oag.state.tx.us/opinopen/opinions/orl50abbott/orl2003/or032162.ht m.

As it turns out, the Maryland banking department also imposed conditions on its approval: among other things, that HSBC conduct regular audits of Household, including for compliance with the (narrow) AGs' settlement; "within 30 days after the findings of each regular audit a copy of the findings will be forwarded to the Commissioner," and that HSBC "honors all present and future judgments, settlements, and regulatory actions taken against [Household], and agrees to take corrective action to assure [Household's] continuing compliance." There are also some conditions regarding the so-called referral-up:

> "that beginning on June 1, 2003 and every quarter thereafter, the Commissioner will be provided with a status report on the alignment of HSBC Bank's and [Household's] product lines and credit policies toward the goal of minimizing customer disparities in products and pricing until implemented; and

> "that by Jane 1, 2003, the Commissioner is provided a copy of the 'competitive review' conducted by [Household] to determine how branch offices of HFC and Beneficial might expand their products; and

> "that by June 1, 2003, the Commissioner is provided with an update of the plan to implement this product expansion initiative to include the development of the risk-based pricing model, training and underwriting and thereafter receive quarterly updates until full implementation."

But what does it matter? HSBC has gotten what it wanted.

58.

At Citigroup, too, the sleaze just continues. Inner City Press is sent documents of a CitiFinancial credit insurance sales training session. The word insurance is never used; it's called "protection." Employees are exhorted to sell as much credit insurance as possible: "Every contact a sales opportunity-- sell the financial solution, the delinquency solution, the protection program. 100% documented presentation of available products is the ONLY ACCEPTABLE Performance level." Becoming more specific, the CitiFinancial presentation states that "Protection sales at maximum level can make or break your effort. One $7500 net personal loan can produce $1,190.91 income in the month booked." That'd be insurance premiums. "PL Insurance sales - $17.00 below criteria.. 84% of objective. EquityPlus Insurance -- $4.70 below criteria.. 62.7% of objective... Total cost of missed insurance income opportunity $3,476,873 -- $46,984 average per branch!" CitiFinancial still measures any credit insurance not sold as a missed opportunity.

"It's legal at electronic stores," one of Citigroup's funkies tells ICP at the shareholders' meeting at Carnegie Hall. Sandy Weill is the only one on stage; most of the speakers suck up to him, including Citi's purported opponents. Money buys you friends; "you are a powerful person," an environmental activist tells Sandy. There must be a better way to fight these practices -- a way more systemic, more global, less craven. That, then, will be the next project. That and another sleazy lender, one also making engines for planes dropping missiles: General Electric. It's in private label cards, but wants to get in deeper. It sends offers of credit, it buys home improvement loans. It wants to bring good things to life, including the Tin Men. Fine then, we will fight. Including using human rights, and also telling stories.

It is a game that is founded on fact: the dream and the need of a house; the foreclosure on the dream. What sharper hook than addiction can keep the money flowing? Arbitrageurs of the global economy study shelter costs and refi flows. The bottom half of the market is more complicated: loans that can never be repaid are nonetheless profitable. The loan are written and rewritten; what can be squeezed out, is. It's not dissimilar to Enron: the losses are hidden by multiple schemes.

Why does the watchers blow the whistle? One arb lays down the law: "I don't care that the company's lying; I don't need to know the truth. As long as I know a bit more than the competition, I can profit." It's the same with Fair Disclosure: those who know of the secret meetings are already a step ahead of Joe Schmo. It requires interested outsiders; it requires a sense of scandal that doesn't ebb and flow with the market. It requires new forms and new intuitions.

59.

The glittering Pacific, the American Dream -- the 21st century will belong to Asia. And there the predatory lenders will be. They salivate to enter China, with its one billion pawns, its mud-brick homes to lend against. Citigroup buys five percent of a bank; HSBC has already got eight. Soon it will be all for sale. And so there the watchers must go. From Sichuan and back; from Xinjiang and New Zealand. The revolving door between the industry and its regulators; the sick flow of money that can still now buy elections -- all of it must change. New songs, new plays, new forms. New ways to bottle wine, and also to sell it. Or to give it away...

60.

Predatory lending has gone mainstream in at least two ways. It affects more and more Americans and is taken overseas. The second way is culture: the time has come for a movie about the Wall Street loan sharks. The Enron scandal is dramatized for television, structured around a romance so its ending can be happy. Does this conform to the structure of the human mind and its hunger for stories? Or is it a way to make individuals, and therefore a one-off, the systemization of fraud?

The script for this story is not in need of fiction. It is not always photogenic: there are dusty fax machines and hours above them; there is legal research and the opening of mail. The documents, however, tell stories of their own. A travel budget, to film it, is required: the expression on the faces of HSBC directors in London and Hong Kong, for example. *Contra* Hollywood, it does not have a neat ending. It is America in the Aughts. The struggle is ongoing, like everything worth doing.

PREDATORY LENDING
Toxic Credit in the Global Inner City

Selective Notes on Sources

For a less cryptic approach, see "Community Reinvestment in a Globalizing World: To Hold Banks Accountable, From The Bronx to Buenos Aires, Beijing and Basle," by Matthew Lee, in *Organizing Access to Capital: Advocacy and the Democratization of Financial Institutions*, Philadelphia: Temple University Press, 2003; another chapter, on international predatory lending, is forthcoming from Praeger.

Ch. 1 - "*HSBC wants to export it*": Wall Street Journal, November 15, 2002, "HSBC Sets $16 Billion Deal for Household International."

Ch. 2 - "*This is called redlining*": see, e.g., ABC News Nightline, April 10, 1995, Transcript # 3621: The Community Reinvestment Act [and Inner City Press/Community on the Move's victories in the Bronx].

Ch. 3 - "*Deutsche Bank is big in this business*": Bureau of National Affairs Banking Daily, June 24, 1999, "Delta Settles With NYS Attorney General."

Ch. 4 - "*the Fed said it would examine CitiFinancial*": 87 Federal Reserve Bulletin 600, September 2001, "Citigroup - European American Bank."

Ch. 5 - "*Gramlich admits there's a problem*": Financial Times, March 26, 2001, Pg. 29, "New Fed Proposals to Curb Growth of Predatory Lending."

Ch. 6 - "*in Edinburgh the Royal Bank of Scotland*": The Scotsman, August 29, 2001, Pg. 1, "Legal Threat to Royal's Mellon Deal;" *see also*, Glasgow Herald, June 3, 2003, Pg. 19, "RBS Citizens Financial Is Accused Over Lending Practices."

Ch. 7 - "*those who blow the whistle*": American Banker, July 10, 2001, Pg. 20, "Another Ex-Worker Cites Citi as Predator."

Ch. 8 - "*Some asked if it would be illegal*": see, e.g., American Banker, April 14, 1998, Pg. 5, Activist Group Opposing Citi-Travelers Merger."

Ch, 9 - "*From the tabloid Daily News*": N.Y. Daily News, April 8, 1998, Pg. 55, "Merger Rivals Emerge: Consumer Groups Draw Line in the Sand."

Ch. 10 - "*Household Finance... bought Beneficial*": see .e.g., American Banker, May 22, 1998, "Household-Beneficial Deal Provokes Activists."

Ch. 11 - "*They call it ROCopoly*": see (only non-Inner City Press report), American Banker, July 12, 2002, Pg. 1, "Another Fed Probe of Citi Subprime Lending Arm."

Ch. 12 - "*Citi bought a new loan shark*": see, e.g., Washington Post, September 7, 2000, Pg. E1, "Citigroup to Acquire Associates First;" "*non-bank GE is also in the mix*": see, e.g., Wall Street Journal, May 9, 2003, Pg. A3, "GE Plans to Move Into a Risky Area: World of Unsecured Personal Loans."

Ch. 13 - "*threatened to sue them if they spoke against Citi*": see, e.g., Houston Chronicle, July 28, 2001, Pg. 4, "Citigroup Hires Legal Big Guns to Warn Employees, Fight Suit."

Ch. 14 - "*complained to the Village Voice*": see, Village Voice, July 15, 1997, Pg. 33. "There is also AIG": New York Times, July 21, 2001, "Third Insurer to Stop Selling Single-Premium Credit Life Policies."

Ch. 15 - "*U.S. Bancorp... ICP raised it*": see, e.g., Omaha World Herald, December 5, 2000, Pg. 14, "N.Y. Group Challenges Firstar-U.S. Bancorp Deal."

Ch. 16 - "*Loan-to-value ratios of 125 percent... were advertised by the Miami Dolphins' Dan Marino*": see, e.g., Sunday Oregonian, February 7, 1999, Pg. B5, "How to Avoid the Risks of Equity Loans."

Ch. 17 - "*When Household bought Benny*": *see, e.g.*, American Banker, June 4, 1998, Pg. 14, "Fewer Beneficial Branches To Close."

Ch. 18 - "*Four hundred dollars to re-write bad loans*": Financial Mail on Sunday, December 29, 2002, "Fresh Row Erupts at HSBC's GBP 9.7 Billion American Bid Target."

Ch. 19 - "*Lehman.com*": *and see*, Financial Times, November 20, 2002, Pg. 24, "Household Acts to Thwart Block on Bid: HSBC Acquisition Threatened."

Ch. 20 - "*It was not Fair Disclosure to play hide-the-ball*": AFX (Agence France Presse), November 28, 2002, "NY Group Urges SEC to Force HSBC to Disclose Household Deal Details."

Ch. 21 - "*ICP retransmits*": *see, e.g.*, American Banker, December 13, 2002, Pg. 1, "Citi Moving Fast to Put Associates Suits to Rest."

Ch. 22 - "*Leah for Sandy has attacked*": *but see*, American Banker, July 30, 2001, Pg. 4, "Citi Corroborates Two Allegations."

Ch. 23 - "*Sir Bond... mistook Mack for Orrin Hatch. ICP raised the issue*": *see*, Business Week Online, November 19, 2002, "HSBC: Why the British Are Coming."

Ch. 24 - "*could have prevented any of the underwriters with bank affiliations*": *see*, Bond Buyer, February 26, 2003, Pg. 36, "Court Delays N.Y.C. Predatory Lending Law So G.O. Deal Can Proceed."

Ch. 25 - "*After she's hired, Inner City Press runs her story*": *and see*, American Banker, October 11, 2002, Pg. 1, "Fed Going Extra Mile In Probe of CitiFinancial."

Ch. 26 - "*the Fed curtly said that its examination is ongoing*": 88 Federal Reserve Bulletin 485, December 2002, "Citigroup - California Federal Bank;" *see also*, Dow Jones Newswires, October 30, 2002, "Fed Expands Citigroup Probe To Insurance-Sale Practices: In Approval of Golden State Purchase, Subprime-Lending Issues Are Detailed."

Ch. 27 - "*the books were being cooked, the loans being 're-aged'*": *see, e.g.*, The Economist, November 23, 2002, "Bottom-fishing."

Ch. 28 - "*began in '92 with the Bank of New York*": Associated Press, September 22, 1992, "A Bank of New York Proposal Hits a Snag;" New York Times, September 23, 1992, Pg. D1.

Ch. 29 - "*challenge to NatWest, for a merger in Jersey*": *see*, Bergen Record, July 30, 1994, Pg. A12, "Bronx Group vs. NatWest: Activists Accuse Bank of Redlining;" Bergen Record, August 24, 1994, Pg. C1, "NatWest to Expand Lending to the Poor."

Ch. 30 - "*fixed a vacant building... legalize other homesteading buildings*": *see, e.g.*, Los Angeles Times, February 27, 1994, Pg. A1, "A Turf War for Urban Squatters;" New York Times, May 31, 1998, "Homesteaders, Nearly Homeowners: After Hard Work and a Break, a Building Is Almost Theirs;" New York Times, September 19, 2002, Pg. F1, "Uptown Settlers Unsettled."

Ch. 31 - "*by afternoon it's on A.P.; it's in the Financial Times*": Associated Press, November 14, 2002, "HSBC to Buy Household International;" Financial Times, November 15, 2002, "Lender With An Unenviable Reputation;" Wall Street Journal, November 15, 2002, "HSBC Sets $16 Billion Deal for Household International."

Ch. 32 - "*It's Eldon who responds*": Reuters, November 20, 2002, "HSBC Hopes Challenges Won't Delay Household Deal."

Ch. 33 - "*Sandy remains, fiddling in his faux-fireplaced office on Park Avenue, ready for all comers*": *see, e.g.*, Business Week Online, June 26, 2002, "King of Capital" [and note that the book by this title exemplifies capitulation, to say the least].

Ch. 34 - "*Why didn't you seek enough money from Household to fully compensate all harmed consumers?*" *See, e.g.*, Albany Times Union, February 3, 2003, Pg. B2, "Complaint Alleges Violations."

Ch. 35 - "*From A.P. in Des Moines comes some news that's not true... the merger is already done*": *see*, Associated Press, December 16, 2002, "Approval Given on Household Settlement."

Ch. 36 - "*Documentation of this loan was sent to HSBC's directors, in Hong Kong, Canada and London*": *see*, *e.g.*, Hong Kong Standard, January 8, 2002, "Group Warns HSBC's Directors over Household Deal."

Ch. 37 - "*speechwriter coined a phrase: a marriage of a premier deposit gatherer*": *see*, *e.g.*, Wilmington (Del.) News Journal, November 15, 2002, Pg. 7B, "HSBC Will Buy Household."

Ch. 38 - "*She defended a bank that Inner City attacked*": Newsday, November 30, 1994, Pg. A32, "About Banks and The Bronx: Fair is Fair."

Ch. 39 - "*Off-color jokes in the Financial Times*": Financial Times, April 30, 2001, Pg. 26, "The Fund Manager and the Porn Star."

Ch. 40 - "*Citi's Number Two Man*": Wall Street Journal, September 10, 2002, "Longtime Adviser to Weill Sits Among Contenders to Throne."

Ch. 41 - "*Household committed*": *see supra* Ch. 10, *and see* Milwaukee Journal Sentinel, June 21, 1998, Pg. 5, "Household to Appease Groups: Opposition to Acquisition Leads to New Loan Terms, Credit Counseling."

Ch. 42 - "*When the day for argument comes*": *see*, American Banker, January 14, 1997, Pg. 1, "Appeals Court Hears Activists' Bid to Sue Fed."

Ch. 43 - "*appeal to the Supremes comes next*": *see*, American Banker, April 8, 1998, Pg. 4, " Docket: Activists to Justices: Allow Court Challenges to Deals."

Ch. 44 - "*It is a lie*": *see*, *e.g.*, National Mortgage News, September 19, 1994, Pg. 14, "NatWest Agrees to Bronx Move After Community Challenge."

Ch. 45 - "*boldly as the Prince down in Dover*": *see*, Wilmington (DE) News-Journal, June 5, 1998, Pg. B7, "Travelers Grilled on Buyout Plan."

Ch. 46 - "*in Singapore... a comment's prepared*": *see*, Straits Times (Singapore) Dec. 31, 2002, "U.S. Group Urges MAS to Pore Over HSBC's Bid for Keppel Insurance."

Ch. 47 - "*venom to Asia... never let it be said the alarm wasn't raised*": *see, e.g.*, Dow Jones Newswires, Dec. 31, 2002, "U.S. Group Urges Monetary Authority of Singapore to Review HSBC / Keppel Deal;" and Financial Times, April 4, 2003, Pg. 18, "Big Lenders Forced to Bank on 'Untouchables' of the Past."

Ch. 48 - "*an application by Option One and its parent H&R Block*"; *see, e.g.*, National Mortgage News, November 25, 2002, Pg. 14, "Community Activists Weigh-In on Household International Buy."

Ch. 49 - "*some fight-back in the works*": *see, e.g.*, Agence France Presse / AFX, November 28, 2002, "NY group urges SEC to force HSBC to disclose Household deal."

Ch. 50 - "*insurance on ladders... lawnmowers, even fishing rods and reels... Inner City asked Sandy about these*": *see*, Wall Street Journal, July 18, 2002, Pg. C1, "Efforts by Citigroup to Reform Subprime Unit Raise Questions."

Ch. 51 - "*staffer from New York:*" *but see*, Origination News February, 2003, Pg. 1, "New York Questions Household-HSBC."

Ch. 52 - "*Charlotte... NationsCredit*": *see, e.g.*, Triangle Business Journal, May 29, 1998, "NationsBank Merger Spurs Probe Requests."

Ch. 53 - "*In Birmingham... their counter-spin*": Birmingham News, July 27, 1999, "AmSouth's lending record criticized."

Ch. 54 - "*phone rates to Warsaw*": *see*, Times of London, January 4, 2003, Pg. 54, "Protesters Target HSBC Directors;" Warsaw Business Journal, January 13, 2003, "HSBC Hunting Kredyt Bank."

Ch. 55 - "*ICP appeals, to the state's Public Access Advisor*": *see*, www.in.gov/pac/advisory/2003/2003fc17.html (visited July 4, 2003).

Ch. 56 - "*a suit in filed in Ohio*": Agence France Presse, March 28, 2003, "HSBC - Household Deal Approval Challenged by Lawsuit Filed by U.S. Consumer Group."

Ch. 57 - "*documents trickle in, even 'post-consummation,' just as they'd planned it*": *see, e.g.*, Hong Kong Standard, March 27, 2003, "HSBC Target Household Accused of Shredding Papers."

Ch. 58 - "*Sandy Weill is the only one on stage; most of the speakers suck up to him*": *see, e.g.*, Newsday, April 16, 2003, Pg. A51, "Activists [at] Citigroup Meeting."

Ch. 59 - "*the watchers must go... New Zealand*": *see, e.g.*, Hong Kong Standard, April 29, 2003, "Advocacy Group Tries to Stop [HSBC-] AMP Deal."

Ch. 60 - "*Predatory lending...is taken overseas*": *see, e.g.*, Financial Times, April 4, 2003, Pg. 18, "Big Lenders Forced to Bank on 'Untouchables' of the Past;" *and see*, chapter, on international predatory lending, forthcoming from Praeger, and "Community Reinvestment in a Globalizing World: To Hold Banks Accountable, From The Bronx to Buenos Aires, Beijing and Basle," by Matthew Lee, in *Organizing Access to Capital: Advocacy and the Democratization of Financial Institutions*, Philadelphia: Temple University Press, 2003.

Off the Clock/Bonus: Global Predatory Lending and How to Fight It

© 2003, Matthew Lee
from a forthcoming work
"Human Rights & Finance"

If the biggest names in finance -- Citigroup, HSBC, General Electric and AIG -- have been engaged in predatory lending in the United States, there's a need for an inquiry into their behavior in less regulated economies beyond the U.S..

An inescapable trend in this new millennium is the export of subprime lending models beyond the United States. Citigroup, following its acquisition of Associates First Capital Corporation in late 2000, began offering subprime loans to lower-income consumers in countries from Brazil and Mexico to India and Korea. The Hong Kong Shanghai Banking Corporation (HSBC) bought Household International a mere month after Household settled predatory lending charges with attorneys general in 42 states for half a billion dollars. In making the deal, HSBC chairman Sir John Bond said that the profits would come from exporting Household's model to the 81 other countries in which HSBC does business (Epstein 2002); a month later, HSBC announced it would compete in subprime with Citigroup in Brazil.

From Australia through North America and back to Eastern Europe, General Electric, through its GE Capital unit, has developed a subprime lending capacity on which the sun never sets. The insurance company AIG has more quietly taken the subprime lending model of American General, which AIG bought in 2001, to the other countries in which AIG goes business.

This consensus around high-rate lending in emerging markets by the world's largest bank (Citigroup), insurer (AIG) and corporation (GE) is indicative of the way in which corporate interests are currently out-stripping (or out-racing) regulation and the public interest. The lenders and their strategies are global, but the laws are at most national, and in some cases state-, county- or merely citywide. In the absence of meaningful regulation, lenders like Citigroup and Household view settlement agreements as a cost of doing business. Both have announced unilateral "best practices" commitments that are applicable by their terms only in the United States (or only in the geographic footprint of the consumers organizations with which they make the announcements). In the short term, there is a need to combat this race to the bottom, similar to anti-sweatshop campaigns and environmental advocacy. In the longer term, there is a need for meaningful global regulation, from a consumer and community point of view, of these emerging global lenders. Related to this inquiry is the view that predatory lending is not *only* a consumer protection and financial soundness issue -- it is also a human rights issue. This argument holds that various nations' signing of, for example, the International Covenant on Economic, Social and Cultural Rights (ICESCR) and the International Convention on the Elimination of All Forms of Racial Discrimination (ICERD) require them to inquire into and act on the predatory lending that exists in, and is being exported into, their countries. Article 2(1)(d) of the ICERD, for example, requires that "[e]ach state party shall prohibit and bring to an end by all appropriate means, including legislation as required by the circumstances, racial discrimination by any person, group or organization." As explored below, and elsewhere, this may be one avenue to pursue accountability in global high-rate subprime lending.

First, however, it is important to inquire into how -- and where, and at what interest rates -- global lenders exported predatory lending in the initial years of the 21st century.

Citigroup has been the leader with this strategy. In acquiring Associates First Capital Corporation in 2000, Citigroup emphasized that the attraction was not only Associates' subprime lending operations in the United States -- according to the Financial Times, "[t]he other principal attraction for Citigroup is Associates' strong presence in Japan, where it can now go head to head with US competitors such as GE Capital." (Hill 2000).

Citigroup and its predecessors were engaged in controversial subprime lending well before the acquisition of Associates in 2000. The upper echelon of management at Citigroup -- outgoing CEO Sandy Weill, incoming CEO Charles Prince, Bob Willumstad, *et al.* -- had all been active with the Baltimore-based subprime lender Commercial Credit, which was challenged for predatory lending in 1997 when it applied to acquire additional subprime business from Bank of America (Timmons 1997) and for a federal savings bank charter (Bell 1997). Based on the protests, filed by Inner City Press / Community on the Move (ICP), the Office of Thrift Supervision agreed to expand nationwide its scrutiny of this subprime savings bank, beyond its Delaware headquarters (Lee 1997). After the 1998 merger with Citicorp

-- in connection with which, Charles Prince was cross-examined about Commercial Credit's lending practices (Epstein 1998) -- Commercial Credit was renamed CitiFinancial; this name was retained and imposed on the controversial Associates business, acquired in late 2000 and then taken global.

By early 2001, it was reported that "Citigroup, the world's largest financial services provider, began its Indian operations with the launch of CitiFinancial Retail Services India Limited. To begin with CitiFinancial will offer easy financing schemes, at retail outlets for the purchase of consumer durable, PC and two wheelers" (India Business Insight 2001).

As with other things at Citigroup, the global expansion of the subprime CitiFinancial was not piecemeal, but rather fully strategized and inexorable. Soon after buying the second-largest bank in Mexico -- a transaction that was widely protested, including by ICP and its new internationally-minded affiliate, the Fair Finance Watch, on the grounds of Citigroup's predatory lending (Lipowicz 2001) -- Citigroup formed what it called a "Consumer Products Unit For Emerging Markets," saying that " the new unit would accelerate the expansion of non-banking consumer financial services into the emerging markets" (Citigroup / Business Wire, May 29, 2002). This press release indicated how and where CitiFinancial was going, by contrasting that "Citibank has consumer-banking operations in 36 of its 80 emerging market countries" with the fact that "[i]n the Emerging Markets Citigroup today has consumer finance businesses in 8 countries with assets of $2.5 billion." And so, onwards!

A major emerging market targeted by CitiFinancial is Brazil. Charging interest rates up to 40%, CitiFinancial in early 2003 opened nine offices in Brazil, projecting that it would open 100 more branches over the next five years (Latin Trade 2003). Regarding this expansion, CitiFinancial Mortgage senior vice president L. Ramesh has been quoted that "[i]n several markets, we are the first ones to give them consumer credit... [We ask:]'Where do you live? What kind of stuff do you have?'" (Bank Systems & Technology 2003).

Inquiring into "what kind of stuff do you have" is reminiscent of CitiFinancial's inquiries with its U.S. personal loan customers, in order to sell them credit insurance they may not need. ICP Fair Finance Watch documented this practice to the Federal Reserve Board, asked then-Citigroup CEO Sandy Weill about it at the company's April 2002 annual meeting; the Wall Street Journal finally got and reported Citigroup's answer:

> When it makes a personal loan, CitiFinancial often asks the holders of personal loans to provide collateral. In some cases, according to CitiFinancial documents filed by Inner City Press, that collateral includes fishing lures and tackle boxes, record albums, tents, sleeping bags and lanterns -- items that CitiFinancial would almost certainly never bother to collect in the event of a borrower's default. Yet insurance is sold on the collateral in case it is damaged or lost.
>
> "It's predatory: This insurance product has no rationale, because it's not credible that someone would want to have their loan paid with their leaf-blower," said Matthew Lee, executive director of the Fair Finance Watch project at Inner City Press. "Citigroup has not lived up to the subprime lending reforms it announced after acquiring Associates."
>
> Citigroup officials concede seizing such collateral would be more hassle than it's worth. But they say providing such collateral on loans has a purpose -- "to make the borrower more responsible for paying the loan back," says Ajay Banga, Citigroup's business head of consumer lending.
>
> (Beckett 2002)

Here, Citigroup acknowledged that while it asked its customers "what kind of stuff do you have?" in order to list the items as collateral and sell insurance on them, it has no intention of foreclosing on the collateral. In fact, Inner City Press has been informed by current and former CitiFinancial employees that the property lists are compiled in order to sell insurance (Mandaro 2002).

Outside of the U.S., not only can insurance be sold -- interest rates of over 25% can be commanded. Since acquiring Associates, EAB and Banamex, CitiFinancial opened in South Korea, charging interest rates of thirty percent. "Although these rates are higher than the annual 24 percent charged by credit card companies for similar cash advances, CitiFinancial has an edge in that their loans are cheaper than those extended by existing loan sharks... Another reason that people are drawn to the company is because of the renowned brand of its parent group, Citigroup. Customers thus tend to think the company will refrain from excessively aggressive collecting methods" (Korea Herald 2002).

The trust that Citigroup would eschew excessively aggressive collection practices, particularly overseas, would be misplaced. The Asian Wall Street Journal, for example, reported on a Citibank loan in India being collected on with no less than a knife to the throat:

> Vikas Dresswala was working in his fabric shop one day in February when three men entered. He says one of them put a knife to his throat and told him: "You give the money now. Otherwise, we'll kidnap you." But this was no robbery. His visitors wanted him to pay his credit-card bills. Mr. Dresswala says he pleaded for time, and the men said they would return in three days, warning that he must pay them then or face the consequences. When they came back, waiting with him were undercover police. "They came in and started threatening," says a police officer, Vanaiak Vast, who says one of the three visitors told the shopkeeper: "I want the money right now or I will kill you."

> The police arrested the three and later accused them of extortion and making terrorist threats . The same accusations were filed against the head of the collection agency, known as Quality Consultants. And the credit-card debt? It was owed to Citibank , the leader of India's surging credit-card market, which had hired Quality Consultants to collect the overdue account (Stecklow and Karp 1999).

This issue was raised to the U.S. Federal Reserve Board, when Citigroup in 2001 applied for regulatory approval to acquire European American Bank (EAB) and Banamex. The Fed's reaction, in its approval orders, was that "claims about lending activities in India... are either outside the jurisdiction of the Board" or "contain no allegations of illegality or action that would affect the safety and soundness of the institutions involved in the proposal, and are outside the limited statutory factors that the Board is authorized to consider when reviewing an application under the [Bank Holding Company] Act." (Fed. Res. Bull. 2001: n.61 (Banamex), n.63 (EAB)).

To jump forward in the inquiry: if the Federal Reserve Board, Citigroup and CitiFinancial's home country supervisor, will not consider CitiFinancial's worldwide compliance practices, who will? The Fed's hands-off approach can be contrasted to the stated jurisdiction of the German regulator, the Bundesanstalt für Finanzdienstleistungsaufsicht, to which ICP Fair Finance Watch directed comments (about GE Capital) in 2003:

> "In the context of our ownership control following section 2b German Banking Act we have to research not only into GE Capital´s business activities in Germany, but also in the USA and worldwide. We consider the information that you delivered on GE Capital´s business practices as important. In a first step, we will request from GE Capital a statement on your concern." (Kallmeyer 2003).

United States government agencies' unwillingness to consider U.S.-based lenders' practices outside of the U.S. leads to a major regulatory loophole, at which other lenders are lining up. As argued below in this chapter, with reference to the failure of U.S.-limited subprime lenders The Money Store (which cost Wachovia over $2 billion) and Green Tree (which drove Conseco into bankruptcy), it may well be that subprime lending confined to the U.S. is a dicey proposition, while taking it overseas to less regulated markets is the industry's future.

This certainly is the business strategy of HSBC, which on November 14, 2002 announced the acquisition of Household International for over $14 billion. A month previously, Household had reached a preliminary settlement of charges of predatory real estate lending and insurance practices with state attorneys general, for $484 million. HSBC seemed unconcerned: the Wall Street Journal reported that Household "could also be rolled out to other countries, HSBC said. 'This is a business we could take to Japan,' HSBC's Sir John said. 'It's already an international business, but we think we could have opportunities in Brazil and Mexico. We haven't examined all the possibilities, but we think they could be extensive.'" (Portanger 2002). The profits, too -- because global subprime lending is subject to few if any restrictions, including self-imposed restrictions. While pressure brought to bear in the U.S. had led Citigroup, AIG and Household to make certain "best practices" commitments in the United States, none has moved to extend these protections anywhere outside of the U.S.. Asked about this, at ICP's initiative, A spokeswoman for HSBC declined to comment" and "Citigroup spokesman Steve Silverman said the company was proud of having 'very good' lending practices throughout the world" (Reckard 2003). But none of Citigroup's commitments are binding, even in the U.S., and the Federal Trade Commission and the class action lawyers in the companion case *Morales v. Citigroup* [San Francisco Co. Super. Ct.] failed to impose any injunctive relief in their $240 million settlements with Citigroup. Meanwhile, as sketched above, CitiFinancial was expanding rapidly overseas, with no committed-to safeguards at all.

When American International Group, Inc. (AIG), the world's largest insurer, applied for regulatory approval to buy American General in 2001, ICP Fair Finance Watch opposed it, noting among other things American General's continued use of single premium credit insurance in connection with its subprime loans. Once ICP raised the issues, AIG's general counsel committed to regulators that single premium credit insurance would be discontinued (McGeehan 2001). Less than two years later, in reporting its first quarter 2003 earnings, AIG let drop that its "growing overseas consumer finance business is performing profitably" (AIG 2003). Needless to say, AIG has not made any best practices or consumer protection commitments in connection with its "growing" non-U.S. consumer finance business.

Another U.S.-based lender which engages in high-rate consumer finance overseas with little oversight is Wells Fargo. Wells' predecessor Norwest was one of the first U.S.-based companies to see the profits possible with a business line targeted overseas and, relatedly, at immigrant groups in the United States. In 1995, Norwest acquired Puerto Rico-based Island Finance from ITT; in announcing the acquisition, Norwest (and now Wells Fargo) CEO Dick Kovacevich said that it portended further "expansion into other Latin American markets (Norwest 1995). Along with Island Finance, Norwest acquired branches in branches in Panama, Aruba, the U.S. Virgin Islands, and the Netherlands Antilles. In 1997, Norwest opened a branch of Island Finance at 2866 Third Avenue in the South Bronx. ICP/Fair Finance Watch's inquiries found that this branch charged 25% interest rates to all customers, without regard to credit history. The office was later closed, and its customers were instructed to travel to a Wells Fargo Financial office in adjacent Queens County to make their payments. In early 1998, Wells purchased a consumer finance company in Argentina, Finvercon S.A. Compania Financiera. Wells also has "Island Finance" subsidiaries in the Cayman Islands, British West Indies, and in Trinidad and Tobago, and operates under the name "Financiera el Sol" in Panama. While its 2000 SEC Form 10-K listed Wells Fargo Financial offices in Brazil, Hong Kong and Taiwan, neither in that SEC report nor elsewhere has Wells made public further information about these stealth, presumably high-rate consumer finance operations.

Wells Fargo is also engaged in controversial high-rate finance in Canada: Wells' "Trans Canada Credit charges 28.9 per cent interest," in the following ways:

> The first thing Labatte did receive appeared to be a credit card statement, showing a limit of $4,150, a billing date of Jan. 23 and a due date of Feb. 23. It stated no minimum payment was owed. Two more monthly statements followed, but Labatte claimed no statements arrived in April or May. He and his spouse both worked and failed to notice the six-month
> deferment period had expired.

> By the time they started making inquiries, a representative of Trans Canada Credit informed them they'd missed the deadline for their "no-interest" offer and now owed approximately $600 in interest payments, dating back to the original date of purchase in November 2002. (MacRury 2003).

This is reminiscent of what is called predatory lending in the United States; Wells Fargo, however, had not included its Canadian or other non-U.S. subsidiaries in what few best practices and/or consumer compliance announcements it has made, despite being pointed asked about this (Reckard 2003).

Similarly, while Household signed consent decrees in over 40 U.S. states in December 2002, HSBC has not committed to any safeguards as it exports Household model overseas. In fact, HSBC's Asia chairman David Eldon has been quoted that HSBC has no problem with Household's past practices (Reuters 2002) -- something that bodes badly for consumers in HSBC's Asian markets. In Brazil as well: a month after HSBC consummated its acquisition of Household, it announced it was exporting subprime consumer finance to Brazil, aiming at a lowest income demographic than CitiFinancial. Dow Jones newswires captured the tit-for-tat, the accelerating global race to the bottom, so to speak, between HSBC and CitiFinancial:

> [HSBC] is launching its own consumer finance operation targeting low-income clients. This comes just weeks after its larger global rival Citigroup Inc. (C) unveiled a similar plan here.... [T]he two global banks are going head to head for the first time in the low-end consumer finance market... [HSBC] looks to conquer 5% to 10% of a 10 to 12 billion-real ($1=BRL2.91) market... [HSBC] plans to launch its new initiative July 1 with the opening of three outlets in Sao Paulo - Brazil's wealthiest city. Within five years, HSBC plans to raise the total to 120 sites for a brand that doesn't yet have a name. The U.K. bank plans to target customers who earn between BRL400 and BRL1,500 a month. The plan, which has been in the works since last year, is similar to that of CitiFinancial The U.S. bank is targeting earners of between BRL500 and 2,000 and wants to set up 100 sites within five years... Consumers pay up to six times higher for credit than the central bank's current reference lending rate of 26.5% and consumer groups have accused them of being greedy. (Dovkants 2003).

But consumer groups' accusations are more nuanced than this. Their indictments include that the companies do not price according to risk, that they strong-arm customers into taking out unnecessary credit insurance of limited value, etc.. But one of the reasons that the new global subprime lenders are focused on non-U.S. markets is due to the under-development to date of consumer protection. For example, GE Capital does retail subprime lending in virtually every continent *but* North America and the U.S.. Beyond GE's acquisition of the U.K. subprime lender First National -- a sort of HSBC / Household in reverse -- GE for example offers high-cost mortgage loans in Australia to "borrowers with court rulings against them" (Kavanagh 2003); GE has been offering subprime loan in Japan "under the 'Honobono Lake' brand" (Japan Economic Newswire 2003). In the subprime consumer finance in the Czech Republic, GE Capital Multiservis is "the largest firm in the field;" its general director Jioi Pathy told the Prague Tribune that "I don't expect any decrease in demand for consumer loans in the near future, because not all of the types of products that are usual in developed economies have been brought to the market yet, and this type of financing is yet to cover all commodities" (Vykoukal 2003). In South Korea, GE Capital is offering prime and subprime loans through kiosks:

> GE Consumer Finance-Korea, a unit of GE Capital Korea, said Wednesday it will offer personal loans via "CashVill" kiosks at two downtown subway stations in Seoul as of Thursday. With the "CashVill" offices opening at Uljiro Ipgu and City Hall subway stations, GE Consumer Finance-Korea will provide unsecured personal loans of between 2 million won (US$1,682) and 15 million won (US $12,615). The interest rate of such products will be based on an individual's credit standing, with loan tenures ranging from one to three years to meet different customer needs.... GE Consumer Finance, a unit of General Electric Company, with US$80 billion in assets, provides credit services to consumers, retailers and auto dealers in 36 countries around the world. (Asia Pulse 2003).

If GE Capital is making consumer loans, many of them subprime, in 36 countries, whose watchdogging this lending? No one, apparently. Unlike even CitiFinancial and HSBC's Household, GE has made no best practices announcements or commitments. It flies under the radar of the Community Reinvestment Act (CRA) in the U.S.: the three banks it uses to make its credit card and store card loans are each "non-bank banks." In 2003, GE Capital bought home equity loans from Conseco / Greentree, but claimed that the volume of loans was too small to require it to convert for a limited purpose credit card bank, with a CRA program limited it the bank's headquarters city, to a broader retail bank. This despite the fact that GE Capital in 2003 began sending out "live checks," personal loan offers with interest rates up to 22 percent (Kranhold 2003). The GE campaign will be one that is, from the beginning, global.

* * *

On HSBC, ICP Fair Finance Watch commented to a dozen countries in Africa, when HSBC moved to acquire the 40% of Equator Bank which it didn't already own. While the expansion of U.S.-style subprime lending is taking place faster in Eastern Europe, Asia and Latin markets like Mexico and Brazil, it will be directed to Africa as well. The manager of bank supervision for the Central Bank of Kenya wrote back to ICP that

> We appreciate the trouble you took to put the long dossier together and will take full cognizance of your warning about the practice of predatory lending. However we are not aware of any intention by HSBC to buy substantial stakes in any bank in Kenya. Thank you very much for your warning. (Ndwiga 2003)

This response became the concluding argument in a subsequent Financial Times analysis piece, which noted that "the biggest banks in the world by market value, Citigroup and HSBC, have become the biggest players in 'subprime' lending," that "JP Morgan Chase has dipped its toe into the subprime waters by buying a credit card portfolio from Providian Financial," and that "[b]ig-time consumer lending is becoming a small world, after all" -- the Financial Times quotes the author that there "is a global financial system, but there is no global regulation." (Silverman 2003).

That *is* the problem, the lack of systemic regulation of this high-rate lending. In the United States, when one jurisdiction passes a law imposing consumer safeguards, many of the lenders adopt a strategy of leaving that jurisdiction for neighboring ones. That took place with the Georgia anti-predatory lending law (until, under pressure from the rating agencies and government-sponsored agencies, Georgia legislature amended its law); the threat, of turning off the "spigot of credit" (that's often the imagery used), has been deployed in New York, New Jersey, Kentucky and elsewhere. It's akin to the race to the bottom of which anti-sweatshop and environmental justice advocates complain: if one nation tries to improve worker protections, for example, the sweatshop contractors simply move to a neighboring (or far away) less-regulated jurisdiction.

The anti-sweatshop / fair labor movement, however, has at least begun to address this problem. It has proposed minimum standards (the specifics of which vary nation to nation); it has applied pressuring leading to global companies like The Gap and Disney having to make global anti-abuse commitments, and submitting to at least some form of outside monitoring. (Schoenberger 2000). The anti-predatory lending /

credit consumer protection movement is years behind, at least in terms of globalizing the movement.

References

American International Group. "News Release: AIG Reports First Quarter 2003 Net Income of $1.95 Billion vs. $1.98 Billion in the First Quarter of 2002," New York: AIG / Business Wire, April 24, 2003

Asia Pulse. "GE Consumer Finance Expands in South Korean Market," Seoul: Asia Pulse, July 2, 2003

Bank Systems & Technology. "CitiFinancial Adopts Lending Model to Emerging Markets," Bank Systems & Technology, April 21, 2003

Beckett, Paul. "Efforts by Citigroup to Reform Subprime Unit Raise Questions," Wall Street Journal, July 19, 2002.

Bell, Allison. "Travelers Unit's Loan Record Hit," National Underwriter, June 23, 1997, Pg. 3

Citigroup. "News Release: Citigroup Forms Consumer Products Unit For Emerging Markets," New York: Citigroup / Business Wire, May 29, 2002

Dovkants, Anthony. " Brazil To Become Battleground For Giants Citigroup, HSBC," Dow Jones Newswires, April 20, 2003

Epstein, Jonathan. "HSBC will buy Household: Purchase Gives Household a Chance to Escape Reputation," Wilmington (De.) News-Journal, November 15, 2002, Pg. 7B

_____. "Travelers Grilled on Buyout Plan," Wilmington (De.) News-Journal, June 5, 1998.

Federal Reserve Board. "Order Approving Acquisition of a Bank" [Citigroup - EAB] Washington, D.C.: 87 Federal Reserve Bulletin 600, 2001.

Hill, Andrew. "Associates Attracts Mixed Reception," Financial Times, September 7, 2000, Pg. 31

India Business Insight. "Citigroup Unveils Easy Buy Scheme," India Business Insight, January 29, 2001

Japan Economic Newswire. " GE Group to Merge Japanese Consumer Credit and Credit Card Arms," Tokyo: Japan Economic Newswire, April 9, 2003

Kallmeyer, Felix. "Response to Comments from Inner City Press / Fair Finance Watch," Bonn: Bundesanstalt für Finanzdienstleistungsaufsicht, June 17, 2003 (on file with the author).

Kavanagh, John. "Money For Non-conformists," Business Review Weekly (Australia), May 8, 2003, Pg. 64

Korea Herald. "Domestic banks forced to sit by as CitiFinancial streaks past," Korea Herald, July 30, 2002.

Latin Trade. "Branching Out," Latin Trade, July 2003.

Lee, Matthew. "OTS Curbs on Travelers' Thrift A Model for CRA in New Era," American Banker, December 10, 1997, Pg. 4.

Lipowicz, Alice. "Predatory Lending Issues Prey on Citi's Banamex Buy: Consumers Want Careful Review Before Deal with Mexican Bank Gets the OK," Crain's New York Business, July 9, 2001, Pg. 4

MacRury, Al. "Know Your Deferred Contract; Buy Now / Pay Later Plans Can Become Costly," Hamilton Spectator, June 26, 2003, Pg. C2

Mandaro, Laura. "Fed Going Extra Mile In Probe of CitiFinancial," American Banker, October 11, 2002, Pg. 1.

McGeehan, Patrick. " Third Insurer to Stop Selling Single-Premium Credit Life Policies," New York Times, July 21, 2001, Pg. C3

Ndwiga, Patrick. "Response to Comments from Inner City Press / Fair Finance Watch," Nairobi: Central Bank of Kenya, February 28, 2003 (on file with the author).

Norwest. "Press Release: Norwest Corporation Completes Purchase of Island Finance Business in the Caribbean," Minneapolis: Norwest / PR Newswire, May 4, 1995.

Portanger, Erik, et al. " HSBC Sets $16 Billion Deal for Household International," Wall Street Journal, November 15, 2002.

Reckard, Scott. "Consumer Group Joins Opposition to Wells Mergers," Los Angeles Times, July 30, 2003.

Reuters. "HSBC Says Hopes to Seal Household Deal as Planned," December 3, 2002

Schoenberger, Karl. Levi's Children: Coming to Terms with Human Rights in the Global Marketplace New York: Atlantic Monthly Press, 2000.

Silverman, Gary. "Household Acts to Thwart Block on Bid: HSBC Acquisition Threatened," Financial Times, November 20, 2002, Pg. 24

_____. "Big Lenders Forced to Bank on 'Untouchables' of the Past," Financial Times (London), April 4, 2003, Pg. 18

Stecklow, Steve and Karp, Jonathan. "Paid Back: Citibank in India Has Hired Collectors Said to Use Threats," Asian Wall Street Journal, May 25, 1999.

Timmons, Heather. "Calling Travelers 'Predatory,'Group Hits Deal with B of A, " American Banker, June 13, 1997, Pg. 3.

Tong, Sebastian. "HSBC's Keppel Bid Opposed," The Hong Kong Standard, January 1, 2003

Vykoukal, Petr. "Leasing: Diversity, Growth and Change," Prague Tribune, June 1, 2003